C000121538

GLUTEN, DAIRY, SOYA, NUT FREE COOKING

GLUTEN, DAIRY, SOYA, NUT FREE COOKING

Nada Farina

NEW HOLLAND

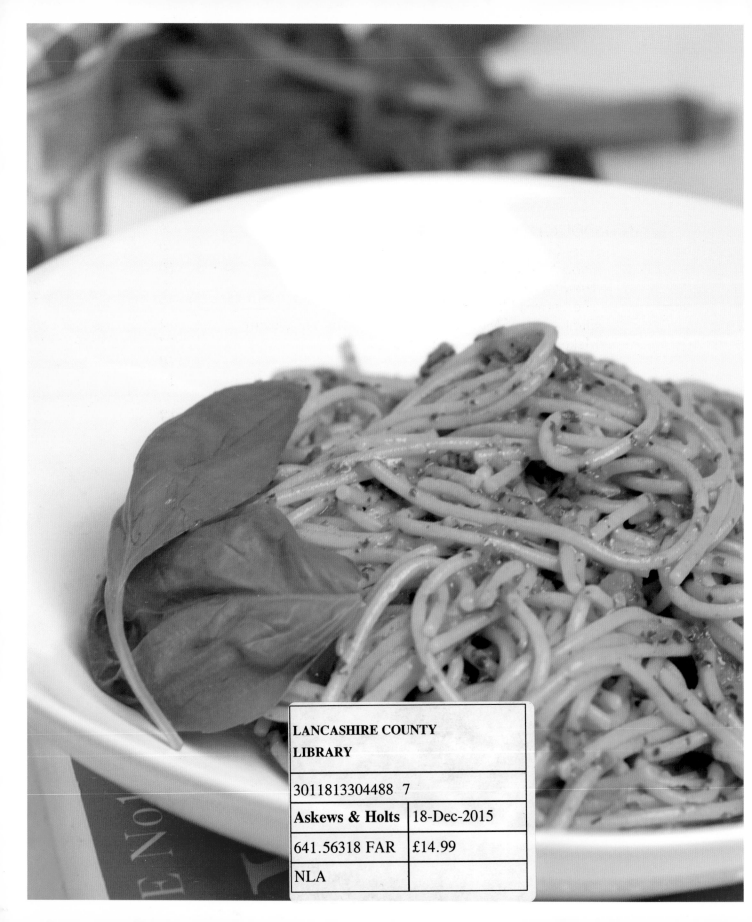

CONTENTS

INTRODUCTION

We all know by now that our diet has a huge impact on our general health and well-being and, deep down, we all know that it is important to be well nourished.

But as the saying goes 'this is easier said than done' taking into consideration our busy lifestyles where we don't always have enough time to cook the food with the freshest, organic ingredients. On the other hand, let's say we had all the time in the world to cook from scratch, it is important to note that we still have a number of other challenges to conquer in order to provide our body with all the essential nutrients. One of the biggest challenges of this kind in today's society is the food hypersensitivity which can be either allergic (food allergy) or non-allergic (food intolerance).

Food allergies or intolerances amongst children and adults are currently at an all-time increase. According to the charity Allergy UK, there are currently around 25 million people in the UK alone suffering from either food allergies or food intolerances. The only prevention for these conditions is an immediate exclusion of one or more offending foods from one's diet. Apart from the food hypersensitivities, there are also other medical conditions, such as Crohn's Disease, Diabetes and Autism that mostly call for an elimination of either gluten and/or dairy.

So, how do we overcome a challenge of food hypersensitivities? Is there a cure? How do we cook and what do we eat/don't eat? These are the first few questions that usually spring into mind any time food allergies are being discussed. These are the questions I was faced with almost three years ago when my first child was diagnosed with food intolerances. This is what prompted me to write this book in the first place. I am really happy to be in a position to share my exciting culinary journey with you and to show you that despite food hypersensitivities, you can still enjoy most if not all of your favorite dishes.

In addition to reinvention of your favorite old classics, you will also be introduced to a number of brand new recipes, all without sacrificing flavor, style or enjoyment.

So, let's learn more about this exciting culinary journey, a journey of gluten, dairy, soya and nuts free cooking.

Almost three years ago I was told that my first child was intolerant to dairy, gluten and soya and that I immediately needed to exclude these allergens from his diet, at first, I was very confused and worried. My first thought was: what is he going to eat now as my cupboards were packed with these allergens? I went to a local supermarket to check their 'free from' food section. In fact, I have quickly realized that most supermarkets have small sections with 'free from' foods but the choice of what to eat is still very limited and even more so in case of multiple food intolerances. To face up to the challenge of not being able to include any gluten, dairy, soya or nuts in my cooking, I knew I needed to make a big change and formulate a healthy diet and lifestyle changes that are sustainable, practical and achievable. And this is exactly what I have done with great support of my husband.

After a new diagnosis, we decided to change our diet as well and eat the same foods as our children so that they did not feel excluded in any way. This was definitely one of the easiest decisions to make.

Having a scientific background with a deeply embedded interest in nutrition and my husband being a 'natural born chef', we have joined our skills and knowledge to create this great collection of high quality dairy, gluten, wheat, soya and nuts free recipes. This book helped us greatly to overcome downsides of the food intolerances and it has also greatly contributed towards the improvement of our own health and well-being. We have definitely introduced more variety of fresh and unprocessed foods into our daily diet, and this sudden transition into the dairy, gluten, soya and nuts free world, over time, became quite easy as well as enjoyable. Every new meal on the table at first had a question mark but then when we all tasted it and when the meal got a seal of approval, a recipe was then added into the book.

My husband comes from a large Italian family where great recipes are passed from generation to generation and where Mamma's cooking rules. Only special people can get hold of these recipes or at least that's what he told me. He just instantly knows how to combine ingredients to get the best flavor and taste. Countless times he would produce an incredibly tasty meal even when the cupboards in the kitchen were almost empty. He taught me how to cook and has greatly inspired my cooking since. We have tirelessly worked together for almost three years on the development of these delicious recipes.

When it comes to cooking, it is important to look into nutritional components of the ingredients used to ensure that our body gets all the essential nutrients it needs to thrive. As we all know, it is possible to create a very tasty meal but with very little health and nutritional benefits. The main focus of this book is to offer you a broad selection of every day meals that are both, incredibly tasty and highly nutritious.

But how do we know what foods we should really eat to achieve optimal nourishment? Which diet should we follow? To answer these questions I have referred to the Eatwell Plate model, which has been issued by the UK Government as the healthy and nutritionally balanced diet that is primarily recommended to all the UK population. In the USA, there is similar model under the name of the American Food Pyramid, which also aims to provide guidance on a healthy and balanced diet.

On the other hand, what happens with reference to our nutrition when we are on a restricted diet such as the one without any gluten, dairy, soya and nuts described in this book? Is it at all feasible then to follow the Eat Well Plate model to achieve a healthy intake of the essential nutrients? This is another topic that this book covers in great detail.

In terms of both, nutrition and cooking, the biggest challenge to start with was to cook without dairies. In the Western world, dairy is still considered to be the main source of calcium, the essential mineral that builds and maintain strong bones and healthy communication between the brain and various parts of the body. Or is it a myth that we only need calcium for strong bones? The book also includes details on our calcium requirements, its best food sources and its overall function in the body.

All the recipes in this book have been designed with all of you in mind: young, old, pregnant, menopausal, middle aged etc.

***

So, whether you need to follow a dairy, gluten, soya and nut free diet because of medical reasons or simply as a matter of choice, or even if you want to cook a nice gluten, dairy, soya and nuts free meal for your special guest, I hope you find this book useful.

ABOUT THIS BOOK

This book brims with imaginative and wonderfully tasty gluten, dairy, soya and nuts free recipes. It aims to encourage you to follow the Eatwell Plate model for a healthy balanced diet that has been officially issued by the UK Government.

It is aimed at:

- All of you who, as a matter of choice, would like to embrace gluten and/or dairy free eating – this diet will not only improve the quality and variety of food you eat by cooking with fresh and unprocessed ingredients but will also improve your energy levels and overall health and well-being when followed correctly. This book is also aimed at those of you who are already following a gluten and/or dairy free diet or would occasionally like to consult a cookbook when cooking for your friends or families that don't eat these foods. This book excludes the following eight out of 14 common allergens: gluten, lupin, milk, mustard, peanuts, sesame seeds, soya and tree nuts.

- Coeliacs and other food allergy and food intolerance sufferers who, for medical reasons, need to eliminate all or any of these four common allergens – gluten, dairy, soya and nuts. Please note that the recipes can be altered if you wish to include any of these allergens into your diet at a later stage.

- People with other conditions and diseases that call for a gluten and dairy free diet such as Autism, Crohn's disease, Diabetes etc.

In today's fast and fake Food World, this book is a real eye-opener as it shows how, with easy to find ingredients and with a touch of imagination and creativity, one can easily prepare incredibly tasty, healthy and nutrition-packed meals even when on a very restricted diet. Today's food industry is still very much dominated by dairy, wheat and, surprisingly soya (according to the charity, Allergy UK, around 60% of all the manufactured foods contain soya) so to cook without all these allergens (gluten, dairy, soya and nuts) was very challenging until now.

All the recipes are designed with our busy lifestyles in mind and are made with easy-to-source ingredients: most are quick and easy to prepare, with many suitable for freezing.

All the recipes have been tasted numerous times before, receiving a seal of approval from my family and friends and only then have they been incorporated into this book.

The good news is that many of our friends didn't taste any difference when dining at our house. Until I told them, they didn't even realize that all the meals they were eating didn't include any gluten, dairy, soya or nuts.

So, if you, your child or anyone you know has been diagnosed with a food allergy or food intolerance, please do not panic. Simply use this book as a guideline for healthy and nutritious eating and choose meals freely according to your own family's likes and dislikes. Also, bear in mind that the number of servings will vary depending upon the ages and appetites around the table. Recipes in this book represent average portion sizes only.

As a family, we have truly enjoyed cooking and even more eating these delicious recipes and I hope you will too.

FOOD ALLERGY OR FOOD INTOLERANCE

We all react differently to different foods. There is no one definite test because food hypersensitivity takes on different forms such as:

- Food allergy – Classical immediate reaction to food(s), which is mediated by IgE antibodies.

- Coeliac disease, which is a reaction to the gluten protein and is detected by measuring anti-tissue transglutaminase (tTGA) and anti-endomysial (EMA) antibodies.

- Food intolerance is non-allergic food hypersensitivity and is not mediated by IgE antibodies. The symptoms of food intolerance generally take longer to emerge when compared to food allergies. Onset typically occurs several hours after ingesting the offending food.

- Enzyme deficiencies such as lactose intolerance.

- Chemical sensitivities such as reactions to food additives e.g tartrazine (E102) and sunset yellow (E110) or other chemicals in foods.

- Reaction to histamine in foods.

It can be difficult to determine whether you have a food intolerance or allergy because often signs and symptoms overlap.

Despite our knowing more than ever about the issues surrounding food allergies and the foods that may cause them, food allergies and food intolerances still remain a complex and challenging matter.

According to the European Food Information Council (EUFIC) the following 14 common food allergens appear to present the most food allergy and intolerance risk and are, therefore, subject to labeling legislation:

Major food allergens
Celery
Cereals containing gluten
Eggs
Fish
Lupin (a kind of legume of the Fabaceae family)
Milk
Molluscs
Mustard
Peanuts
Sesame seeds
Shellfish
Soya
Sulphur dioxide (used as antioxidant and preservative, e.g. in dried fruits, wine, processed potatoes)
Tree nuts

Please note that the recipes in this book do not include any: gluten, lupin, milk, mustard, peanuts, sesame seeds, soya and tree nuts but they do include eggs, celery, fish, mollusc, shellfish and sulphur dioxide (from dried fruits only).

THE EATWELL PLATE

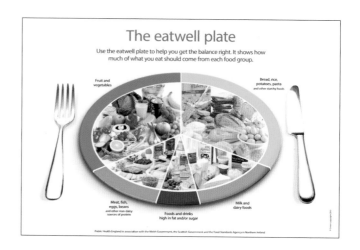

*The Eatwell Plate image is subject to Crown copyright protection, which is covered by an Open Government Licence. It has been issued by Public Health England in association with Welsh Assembly Government, the Scottish Government and the Food Standards Agency in Northern Ireland.

This book is based on the Eatwell Plate model that has been officially issued by the UK Government to define government's advice on a healthy balanced diet.

According to the Public Health England, the Eatwell Plate is a visual representation of how different foods contribute towards a healthy balanced diet and is appropriate for all healthy people over two years of age.

The Eatwell Plate is based on five food groups and shows how much of what you eat should come from each food group. This includes everything you eat during the day, including snacks.

- Plenty of **fruit and vegetables** (at least five portions a day).

- Plenty of **potatoes, bread, rice, pasta and other starchy foods**.

- Some **milk and dairy**.

- Some **meat, fish, eggs and/or non-dairy sources of protein**.

- Only a small amount of **high fat/or sugar foods**.

It also is not necessary to follow the model rigidly at every single meal – instead, it is recommended to get the balance between the different food groups right over a longer period of time. Most of what we eat should come from ingredients shown in the two biggest food groups – starchy foods, fruit and vegetables. The meat, fish, eggs, beans group and the milk and dairy products group are smaller, illustrating that quantities from these groups should be less. Only occasional or limited intakes of foods high in fat and/or sugar are signalled by this being the smallest section as these foods are not essential to a healthy diet. Each of the four main groups provides a different range of essential nutrients, emphasising the importance of a varied diet. The Eatwell Plate does not include reference to frequency of serving and recommended portion sizes, other than in relation to fruit and vegetables such as at least five portions of variety a day. The key messages about a healthy diet, as depicted in the Eatwell Plate, are about eating a variety of foods to achieve the range of nutrients we need for a healthy lifestyle and eating the right amount of food for our weight. The segments of the plate represent the proportion the food group should make towards the whole diet. We differ in the amount of energy (calories) we require and that affects the amount of food, in total, individuals need.

All the recipes in this book have been analyzed with the Eatwell Plate in mind. The Eatwell Plate has been represented in a pie-chart format, showing recommended proportions of five food groups. Most of the recipes contain the first four food groups, so simply by cooking and introducing those meals into your daily diet, you will ensure that your body is optimally nourished.

THE EATWELL PLATE AND FOOD INTOLERANCES

The Eatwell Plate Model and Food Allergies and Intolerances do not exactly go hand in hand. The Eatwell Plate model calls for a balanced and varied diet including all the main food groups while the Food Intolerances and Allergies call for an elimination of certain foods or even food groups. But, how do we deal with this issue?

The best way to decide what to do is to first know how much or what vitamins and minerals are required for your body, then learn which replacement foods contain those vitamins or minerals. So, if it sounds feasible for you to eat those foods every day, then your problem is already solved here. But, if you can't imagine that you could eat or prepare all the necessary foods each day, then it is advisable to ask your doctor to prescribe you some supplements depending on your food sensitivities.

Once my children were diagnosed with food intolerances to dairy, gluten, soya and nuts, at first, I knew it was going to be very challenging to be able to offer them foods containing all the essential vitamins and minerals on a daily basis. The truth is there are many products now available in the supermarkets that are either dairy or gluten free but hardly ever dairy and gluten and soya free. Interestingly, most of the people nowadays incorrectly assume that if you are intolerant to dairy that you can actually tolerate soya.

Recent research has shown that if you are intolerant to a milk protein in cow's milk, then there is around 80% chance that you are intolerant to soya protein as these two proteins are similar in structure. The fact that 60% of all the manufactured goods contain soya made it even more difficult to be able to buy any convenience meals in the supermarkets.

This is why in our family there always had to be time for cooking as if not, everyone would be hungry and unhappy. When cooking at home, it is also very important to pay proper attention to the alternative food choices to ensure that we get all the required vitamins and minerals on a daily basis.

As far as the alternative food choices are concerned, food intolerance to gluten and nuts did not present much of a problem, as there are many alternatives that would provide you with all the essential vitamins and minerals. Cooking without nuts at home for my family was not an issue either as it is not difficult to create recipes without any nuts.

Likewise, if you need to eliminate gluten there is a very wide choice of other suitable grains and flours that you can use such as maize, quinoa, rice, chick pea, coconut, hemp, buckwheat, chestnut and the list goes on. Or you can simply use readily available wheat-free gluten free flours.

However, food intolerance to dairy as well as soya has proved to be extremely challenging as there is still a limited choice of ready available products that are both, soya and dairy-free. This is probably due to the earlier mentioned misconception that intolerance to dairies can be overcome by consuming products made from soya.

As far as the Eatwell Plate is concerned, by eliminating milk and dairies from your diet, you are actually eliminating one whole food group from this balanced and healthy eating model. Luckily, nowadays there are many dairy milk alternatives that are already fortified with calcium such as rice or coconut milk that you can use instead.

ELIMINATION OF MILK AND DAIRY – THE QUESTION OF CALCIUM

A dairy- and gluten free diet requires careful consideration and planning to ensure we receive all the nutrients we need to thrive. It is a common belief in the Western World that we need to drink cow's milk and eat dairy products in order to get enough calcium on a daily basis.

Calcium is vital for growth and maintenance of strong bones, teeth and cell walls and has a role in muscular contraction, blood clotting and immunity. In fact, 99% of the body's calcium is found in the bone and teeth. The most crucial time to build strong bones is during childhood and the teen years to avoid osteoporosis later in life.

However, it is important to note that calcium does not work alone. It must have other vitamins and minerals present to function. Calcium works with phosphorus, potassium, sodium, magnesium, and vitamins A, C and D. And only when all these vitamins and minerals are present in our body, calcium utilization and absorption can take place.

Firstly, lets see how much calcium we all need on a daily basis.

Daily calcium intake requirement according to age and as recommended by the National Osteoporosis Society, is as follows:

Age	Daily Calcium Intake
0–12 months	520 mg
1–3 years	350 mg
4–6 years	450 mg
7–10 years	550 mg
11–14 years	800 mg
Teenagers	1000 mg
Pregnant and Nursing Mothers	1200 mg
Males 20–60 years	1000 mg
Females 20–45 years	1000 mg
Females over 45 years	1500 mg
Males over 60 years	1500 mg

Elimination of dairies does not actually mean that getting enough calcium in your diet is impossible. It just means that we need to pay attention to the alternative non-dairy calcium-rich foods as well as combining these with our favorite foods all day long. Also, to help facilitate absorption of calcium, it is imperative that we are getting a daily requirement of vitamins D, C and A as well as potassium, phosphorus and magnesium.

If you are unable to take time to do this, then, it is likely that you or your child will need vitamin as well as mineral supplements. If in any doubt, always seek advice from a relevant medical professional.

The following are non-dairy sources of calcium:

Food	Calcium content per 100 g/100 ml
Almonds	240 mg
Apricots	92 mg
Brazil Nuts	78 mg
Calcium-enriched bread	240 mg per thick slice
Calcium-enriched soya milk, oat milk, hemp milk, coconut milk, almond milk, hazelnut milk	120 mg
Chick peas (raw)	160 mg
Currants	53 mg
Figs (dried)	250 mg
Hazel Nuts	140 mg
Instant calcium-enriched porridge 40g made with calcium enriched plant/nut milk	600 mg
Okra	160 mg
Orange juice with added calcium	100 mg
Parsley	200 mg
Red kidney beans	100 mg
Sesame seeds	670 mg
Soya beans (raw)	240 mg
Spring greens	75 mg
Tahini	680 mg
Tofu	510 mg
Treacle (black)	500 mg
Watercress	170 mg

*Please exclude soya and/or nuts or any other allergens if they cause intolerance.

Most of the dishes in this book contain calcium-rich ingredients.

MAKE TIME FOR MEALS WITH YOUR CHILDREN

Apart from providing your child with good nutrition, it's equally important to make time for meals with your children, even more so if your child is intolerant or allergic to certain foods. One golden rule to remember here is that you want to raise a confident child that does not feel excluded or different than their peers, just because he/she does not eat gluten or drink cow's milk.

As previously mentioned, once my children were diagnosed with the food intolerances, my husband and I decided to change our eating habits and always eat what they eat at home. This book proves that with good organisation skills and creativity, this is not a difficult task. For instance, you can still enjoy your favorite food even when it excludes big allergens such as gluten and dairy.

By eating what your child eats, you are creating a comforting home environment and you are avoiding many upsetting situations when he or she asks and wants foods they can't have. If those foods are not in the house, especially when your children are too little to understand their condition, then it significantly reduces the overall level of stress to your child and you. Not only that, the ritual of regular meals is comforting to our children, it also develops their language and conversational skills, proper table manners and provides opportunities for good nutrition.

Obviously, when your child goes to a nursery, school or to social gatherings, it is of a paramount importance to ensure that all the foods they eat are allergens free. Although nurseries and schools have plenty of experience in handling food allergies and intolerances and many of them provide catering for those children, it is still important to advise them well in advance of your child's intolerances and ask them if they can serve a similar allergen-free version for your child too. If not, it is worth enquiring about the school's menu in advance so that you can prepare food at home that resembles the food that all the other children will be eating in a school or nursery setting. You can label it as a 'special' food for your child. It is an extra effort but it really is worth it. For instance, if all the children in school are having a beef lasagne, there is no reason why your child will need to eat baked potatoes and beans, for example. You can create a version of a dairy or/ and gluten free beef lasagne in the comfort of your own home just by looking at the recipe at page 95.

Likewise, if your child is attending a birthday party, you need to inform the host of your child's intolerances in advance and do not be ashamed to offer an allergen-free selection of food so that your child again does not feel excluded. Most hosts will then go ahead and include a few allergen-free options so that your child can have a meal too. As far as the cake is concerned, this is a difficult one to overcome as all cakes nowadays are loaded with milk products and gluten.

Of course, you cannot expect a host to have a dairy and/or gluten free cake just to accommodate your child, but you can prepare some allergen-free treats at home and send them with your child to a party so he/she can share it with other kids. I usually make dairy- and gluten free chocolate lollipops for my children so they can share them out at the party and it works well each time. Obviously, when the children are older, it is easier for them to understand how to manage their food allergies and intolerances.

The truth is most of us nowadays have busy lifestyles, be it a work commitment or simply household daily chores, so that sitting down and eating together with our children does not happen as often as we would like to. But, dining together as a family should be our top priority whenever possible, even more so if your child is intolerant or allergic to certain foods.

FOOD LABELS

There is currently no cure for food allergy or food intolerance, but the good news is that both conditions can easily be managed by an immediate exclusion of allergen (s) from one's diet. This is why everyone with food intolerances need to pay attention to what they eat or drink at all times.

For instance my children currently lead a normal, happy life since dairy, gluten, soya and nuts have been cut out from their diet. In other words, if they do not consume any of these four allergens, they do not have any problems at all.

Of course, you still need to be very careful when buying all the pre-packaged foods – you really need to pay special attention to all of the food labeling information. And even if you buy the same products over and over again, always check the ingredients list as manufacturers very often decide to change ingredients of the products for various reasons.

According to the Foods Standard Agency in the UK, manufacturers need to label any of the 14 regulatory food allergens in all pre-packaged goods. Manufacturers often use phrases such as 'may contain' to show that there could be small amounts of allergen for example milk, gluten, nuts etc. in a food product because it has entered the product accidentally during the production process.

It is important to understand that different manufacturers can choose to use different phrases to warn of allergen cross contamination risks, such as:

- May contain...

- Made on equipment that also processes...

- Made in a factory that also handles...

These different phrases describe how the risk arises, but are not indicative of the severity of the risk. For this reason, none of these warnings should be read as being more or less serious than another phrase.

So, the best advice here is to always carry your prescribed allergy-rescue medication with you and ensure that your friends and family know how to use it on you.

As the saying goes, prevention is always better than a cure; even more so when there is no cure like in the case of food hypersensitivities.

HOW TO USE THIS BOOK

All the recipes in this book are free from gluten (GF), dairy (DF), soya (SF), lupin, mustard, peanuts, sesame seeds, and tree nuts.

Every dish includes the 'Eatwell Plate' pie chart to indicate the food groups found in that dish. As our individual requirements are different, this book and the Eatwell plate tool itself do not include reference to frequency of serving and recommended portion sizes. To make healthy choices, you will need to identify the main food groups in your meals and think about how these fit with the proportions shown in the Eatwell Plate.

A diet in line with the Eatwell Plate will provide you with all the nutrients and energy that you need. Hence, it is recommended that the EatWell plate diet is followed on a daily basis. This book provides a clear guidance on which foods to include in your diet. Simply by looking at the Eatwell Plate pie chart, you can clearly ascertain which food groups are included in a dish and which ones are missing, if any. There are a number of recipes that include all of the food groups but the ones that don't, need to be supplemented with other foods in order to comply with the Eatwell Plate diet. For instance, if the Eatwell Plate chart shows that a dish contains only proteins and vegetables, this straightaway gives you an indication that you need to include carbohydrates (i.e. a bread roll) and dairy alternatives (i.e. a glass of dairy-free milk) to have a nutritionally balanced die. It is not necessary to follow the model rigidly at every single meal – instead, it is recommended to get the balance between the different food groups right over a longer period

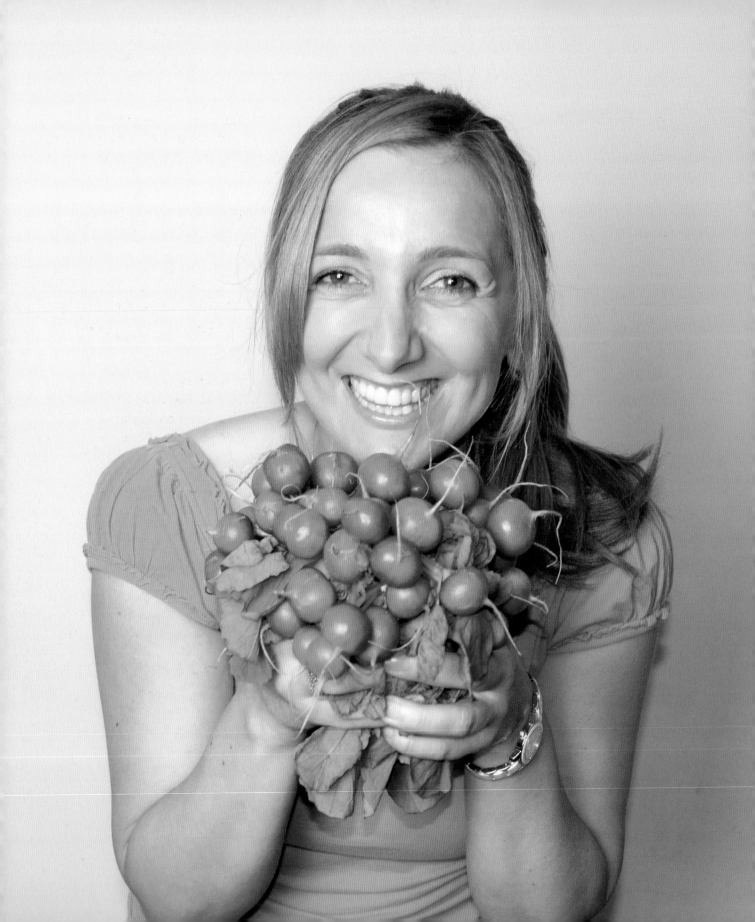

of time. Many dishes in this book already include all of the food groups (fruits and/or vegetables, carbohydrates, proteins and dairy alternatives) hence, by cooking those dishes you are already including all of the essential nutrients into your diet. If a dish contains vegetables but not fruits, please also add a fresh piece of fruit to that meal or vice versa.

Likewise, if a dish is high in sugar and/or fat content, even if it does contain all other food groups, such dish should still be eaten in moderation due to its high sugar and fat content. For instance, all the desserts in this book fall under this category.

The high in sugar and/or fat category has been included in the Eatwell Plate model as most of us do eat those foods. It is important to point out that it is fine to occasionally have a little treat as long as these 'treats' are eaten very occasionally and in strict moderation as they do not fall under a healthy diet umbrella.

The recipes in this book are divided into chapters according to the kind of thing you want to eat. There is also a very good selection of vegetarian as well as vegan options. These recipes show average portion sizes only. Unless otherwise stated, always use fresh, preferably organic, ingredients. Also, use medium eggs, fruits and vegetables and do not mix metric and imperial measurements.

Now that we know what this book is about and how to use it, let's have a look at the ingredients and its nutritional and health benefits.

INGREDIENTS

The quality of the ingredients you buy greatly influences the nutrient content of the food you eat. Whenever possible, the recipes in this book call for fresh organic fruits and vegetables, organically reared meat, wild fish, organic or free range eggs, wholemeal rice and gluten free flours.

This section outlines nutritional and health benefits of all the ingredients used in preparing the recipes in this book. I hope that this will, not only further broaden your knowledge of the food nutrition, but will help you to easily decide what to cook and why. So many times, before I decided to study nutrition, I would eat let's say tomatoes or beetroot without really knowing all the nutritional and health benefits that they provide. And not so many times was I thinking about eating asparagus until I have learned about how good this vegetable really is for our health. Overall, I hope you enjoy reading about the different ingredients and all the nutritional and health benefits they provide. There are many interesting facts that you might not know about:

VEGETABLES

Asparagus
Asparagus is low in calories and is very low in sodium. It is a good source of vitamin B6, calcium, magnesium and zinc, and a very good source of dietary fiber, protein, beta-carotene, vitamin C, vitamin E, vitamin K, thiamin, riboflavin, rutin, niacin, folic acid, iron, phosphorus, potassium, copper, manganese and selenium, as well as chromium, a trace mineral that enhances the ability of insulin to transport glucose from the bloodstream into cells. The amino acid called asparagine gets its name from asparagus, as the asparagus plant is relatively rich in this compound. Asparagine is known to increase urinary output and hence, is useful in conditions such as high blood pressure and fluid retention. Asparagus also has mild anti-inflammatory activity as it contains a chemical called racemofuran.

Avocados
Nutrient-packed avocados are the perfect food for young children. They are rich in energizing B vitamins and monosaturated fats, which are easily digested. Oleic fatty acid in avocados is also found in olive oil and is responsible for the reduction of bad (LDL) cholesterol, and a subtle increase of good (HDL) cholesterol. Avocados are also high in protective antioxidants, including vitamins A, C and E. These antioxidants help protect skin cell membranes from damage maintaining healthy skin. The high vitamin E content of avocados is beneficial for heart health too. Vitamin E is also known as a natural anticoagulant as it reduces blood-clotting activity in the body and, hence, helps prevention of strokes and heart attacks.

Beans

All beans are naturally very high in protein and fiber – a good combination that helps stabilize blood sugar levels and as high fiber food, promote a healthy digestion. Being a useful source of iron, beans can help to avoid anaemia and fatigue. They are also a good source of manganese, zinc and magnesium minerals. Common varieties of beans include black beans, kidney beans, lima beans, navy beans, pinto beans, white beans and chickpeas. White beans can help to maintain strong bones as they are high in calcium. Chickpeas and lima beans are high in zinc, folate, magnesium and vitamin B6. Kidney beans help prevent and manage arthritis, as they are high in vitamin C, an antioxidant that is responsible for production of collagen, a component of cartilage. Kidney beans are rich in magnesium and contain niacin, that may prevent cataracts.

Beetroot

Beetroot is naturally high in iron and folic acid and is, therefore, well known as a blood-boosting food – it helps in production of red blood cells and hence, prevents anaemia and fatigue. Folic acid also helps in lowering homocysteine – a toxic chemical that has been linked to many chronic conditions, including pour mental health. Beetroot is also high in natural nitrates, a type of mineral salt that the body converts into nitric oxide. Nitric oxide is naturally produced to regulate blood pressure. The purple color pigment in beetroot called betacyanin is known to increase the level and activity of detoxification enzymes found in the liver.

Broccoli

Broccoli's nutritional profile is impressive and, hence, they are one of the well-known superfoods. Broccoli contain high levels of powerful pytonutrient antioxidants such as sulphoraphane and indoles, as well as beta-carotene, which can help protect against cell damage, support liver function and promote a healthy respiratory tract and skin. There is also an enzyme in broccoli called myrosinase, which can reduce the risk of developing cancer. However, broccoli should not be overcooked as overcooking will undermine beneficial effects of this enzyme. Therefore, to really get the most out of this vegetable, broccoli should only be lightly steamed rather than boiled. Broccoli is also a good source of iron and folic acid, which is important for haemoglobin production and healthy red blood cells. They also contain high levels of fiber and are a rich source of vitamin C, A, K, B-complex vitamins, zinc, and phosphorus.

Butternut Squash

Butternut squash naturally contains a high level of fat-soluble antioxidants called carotenoids, which give butternut squash a bright orange flesh. Lutein and zeaxanthin carotenoids are essential nutrients for insuring healthy eyesight. Carotenoids also have anti-inflammatory activity and can help to reduce redness of lesions such as acne and eczema and also help to reduce heart disease by reducing the oxidation of fatty compounds such as bad (LDL) cholesterol, which can damage the blood cells. It also contains soluble fiber and is a good source of vitamin B6 and folate, which are important for the production of neurotransmitters in the brain and maintaining a healthy nervous system. Butternut squash also contains high levels of vitamin A, which is a powerful natural anti-oxidant and helps to support the immune system and overall mucosal health.

Carrots

Carrots are excellent for children's immune systems and skin health. They naturally contain high levels of vitamin A, vitamin C as well as calcium and iron. They also contain fiber, vitamin K, potassium, folate, manganese, phosphorus, magnesium, vitamin E and zinc. They contain a variety of antioxidants lending them their color: (beta carotene gives carrots their bright orange color, anthocyanin gives them purple color, lycopen red etc). Beta-carotene is absorbed in the intestine and converted into vitamin A during digestion. It naturally diffuses into fatty tissues such as those in the skin where it can offer antioxidant protection and anti-inflammatory activity making it ideal for conditions such as acne and eczema. Beta-carotene also accumulates in the eyes offering protection from free radical damage, which may help to protect against cataracts. As far as the immune system is concerned, carrots are responsible for the production of T cells in the digestive tract, which help the immune system to fight off infections.

Celery

Celery contains high levels of antioxidant nutrients, including vitamin C, beta carotene, and manganese. Celery also acts as an effective natural painkiller as it contains a compound called 3-n-butylphthalide (3NB for short). It also has anti-inflammatory properties as it contains pectin-based polysaccharides which help to improve stomach lining, decrease risks of stomach ulcers as well as improve the control of stomach secretions. Celery also contains other complex components such as coumarins that help protect against urinary tract infections and high blood pressure.

Chickpeas

Chickpeas are rich in dietary fiber, proteins, vitamin B6, copper, manganese, selenium and calcium. They help to maintain a healthy heart, good blood pressure and are known to lower cholesterol.

Cauliflower

Cauliflower is rich in dietary fiber, vitamin C, vitamin K, vitamin B6, potassium and manganese. It's also a good source of protein, and magnesium and is very low in saturated fats and cholesterol. Cauliflower also has anti-inflammatory properties and is an excellent source of antioxidants.

Eggplant

Eggplants (also known as aubergine) are packed with antioxidants, phenolic compounds, such as caffeic and chlorogenic acid, and flavonoids, such as nasunin. Nasunin has been shown to protect the fatty coating of nerve cells from damage whilst chlorogenic acid has a range of health benefits, including being antimicrobial and ant-viral. Eggplant is very low in calories and fats but rich in soluble fiber content hence, can help to ease constipation. It also contains good amounts of many essential B-complex groups of vitamins such as pantothenic acid (vitamin B5), pyridoxine (vitamin B6) and thiamin (vitamin B1), niacin (B3) as well as minerals manganese, copper, iron and potassium.

Jerusalem Artichokes

Jerusalem artichokes are an excellent source of iron. They are also a good source of thiamine, phosphorus and potassium. They are one of the finest sources of dietary fiber and they also contain small amounts of antioxidants. This root vegetable is eaten in the same way as potato in many parts of Western Europe and Mediterranean regions.

Kale

Kale is very high in calcium, phosphorus, iron and vitamins A, C and K. Being rich in calcium and phosphorus, this vegetable is a great support for skeletal health. Per calorie, kale has more iron than beef. Iron is essential for good health, such as the formation of haemoglobin and enzymes, cell growth, proper liver function etc. Research has shown that Vitamin K can help protect against various cancers. The dark green color of kale indicates that this vegetable is incredibly rich in chlorophyll that contains magnesium. Calcium and magnesium work in tandem in muscle tissue. Calcium causes muscles to contract, whereas magnesium causes it to relax. Kale also contains powerful antioxidants such as carotenoids and flavonoids.

Onions

Onions are naturally high in quercetin – a powerful antioxidant that can help reduce inflammation and lower histamine, making it beneficial for children with allergies. They also contain chromium, which assists in regulating blood sugar levels. Raw onions encourage the production of good cholesterol (HDL), thus keeping the heart healthy. Onions are also rich in inulin which is a potent prebiotic which provides support for digestive health. Consumption of onions results in increased numbers of 'good' bacteria, which are important for good digestion.

Peas

Peas are a good source of protein and fiber and rich in Vitamin C, iron, thiamine, folate, phosphorus and potassium. The high fiber and protein content is beneficial as it helps to slow down digestion of sugars. Furthermore, their antioxidant and anti-inflammatory characteristics may help to prevent or reverse insulin resistance (type 2 diabetes). Research has shown that green peas are a reliable source of omega-3 fat in the form of alpha-Linolenic acid (ALA).

Peppers

Peppers naturally contain many phytochemicals that have antioxidant abilities. They come in a rainbow of colors including green, red, yellow, orange, purple and each color is associated with a different family of phytochemicals. Red peppers contain high levels of vitamin C, vitamin E, beta-carotene and zinc that help support the immune system. They are a good source of fiber, folate, vitamin K and the minerals molybdenum and manganese as well as some B complex vitamins, calcium, phosphorus and iron. Carotenoids present in peppers are also vital for healthy eyesight.

Potatoes
Naturally high in complex carbohydrates, and include both protein and fiber, they provide plenty of sustained energy as well as vitamins B6 and C, iron and potassium. B6 is vital for the production of neurotransmitters including serotonin, which can help to boost our mood. New potatoes when eaten with a skin help to increase our fiber intake and they also release their sugars slowly into the bloodstream hence avoid sudden changes in the body's energy levels. Potatoes also contain a compound called kukoamine, which has been shown to cause a reduction in blood pressure.

Spinach
Naturally high in iron, vitamin C, vitamin B6, calcium, potassium, folate, zinc, and thiamine, it's also packed with a fat-soluble antioxidant beta carotene that may help to protect collagen and elastin fibers from damage.

Sweet Corn
Sweet corn is an excellent source of folate. It also contains good levels of B vitamins, iron, zinc, magnesium, copper and manganese. Sweet corn is rich in the antioxidant called ferulic acid, which plays a vital role in preventing some cancers, aging and inflammation in humans.

Sweet Potato
Sweet potatoes are rich in beta carotene, the substance that is responsible for their bright orange color. Beta-carotene is converted by the body into vitamin A, which has anti-viral and skin protecting properties. Sweet potatoes are also high in fiber, vitamin C, vitamin E, potassium and provide plenty of sustained energy.

Tomato
Tomatoes contain high levels of vitamin C and are also a good source of vitamin E, beta-carotene, magnesium, calcium and phosphorus. They also contain a lycopene, a carotenoid, which is responsible for their red color. It is also an essential antioxidant, which helps to protect skin from UV damage, reducing the risk of cancers by protecting cells and tissues from free radical damage.

Zucchini
Zucchinis (also known as courgettes), are naturally high in soluble fiber and also have a high water content making them an ideal food in the case of constipation. They also contain B vitamins,

including folate, which is important in cell divisions and DNA synthesis. Zucchinis are rich in lutein and zeaxanthin (eye supporting carotenes) that support good eye health. They are also a very good source of potassium, which is a heart friendly electrolyte that helps reduce blood pressure and heart rates by countering pressure-effects of sodium. In addition to B vitamins, they also contain vitamin C, vitamin A as well as minerals: iron, manganese, phosphorus and zinc.

SEAFOOD

Anchovies
Anchovies contain high levels of omega-3 fatty acids that help maintain healthy cholesterol levels and offer protection against damage to the blood vessel walls caused by inflammation. These fats are vital in managing all inflammatory conditions such as asthma, eczema, and arthritis. Anchovies are a good source of calcium, vitamin D, magnesium, and phosphorous which are essential for bone mineral density. They also contain vitamin A, which plays an important role in vision, bone growth, reproduction and cell division.

Cod
High in protein and easily digestible for children, it is also very low in saturated fat and a good source of selenium, and B vitamins, which can aid skin health and support a healthy immune system. Cod is also a good source of iodine, which is essential for thyroid function and metabolism. It also contains phosphorous which helps to form DNA and the haemoglobin in red blood cells.

Mackerel
Mackerel is rich in omega-3 fatty acids, proteins, vitamin D and potassium. It helps to control blood pressure, lowers risk of diabetes and improves cognitive function.

Monkfish
Monkfish is a good source of protein and naturally contains vitamins B6 and B12 that aid in the synthesis of neurotransmitters needed for brain function. It also contains phosphorus and selenium. Selenium controls protein activity and acts as an antioxidant while phosphorous strengthens your children's bones. Monkfish is also low in saturated fat and sodium.

Prawns
Naturally rich in immune supporting minerals, especially zinc and selenium and a good source of omega-3 fatty acids. Omega-3 fatty acids are important for a child's brain development and also help to maintain a healthy immune system and healthy skin. Prawns are rich in astaxanthin, which

gives them their distinctive pink colour and offers some anti-inflammatory activity. Hence prawns are a good choice for children as well as adults that suffer from eczema, acne or psoriasis.

Salmon

Salmon is one of the healthiest foods for your child's brain. It is naturally rich in omega -3 fatty acids that support brain function, help maintain healthy cholesterol levels and protect the blood vessels from inflammatory damage (useful for eczema, psoriasis or acne). Salmon is also a great source of protein, supporting growth and development and to stabilise blood sugar levels through the day. Recent research has shown that omega-3 fatty acids can be beneficial in mental health.

Squids

Squids are a very good source of protein and are low in saturated fats and sodium. They also contain copper, selenium, vitamin B12, riboflavin, zinc, niacin and phosphorus. Niacin is important for metabolism, while B12 is important for red blood cell production and nervous system health.

Tuna

Naturally rich in omega-3 fatty acids, Tuna has the same omega-3 benefits as salmon and sardines. It is very high in selenium, which has proved beneficial for the health of the skin as an anti-inflammatory.

MEAT

Beef

Lean beef is a good source of protein, iron and B vitamins. It is also rich in zinc, which is important for wound healing and immune support. B vitamins are essential for the production of neurotransmitters, which are essential for brain function and memory. Beef also contains vitamin A, riboflavin, niacin, folate, phosphorus, copper and selenium.

Chicken

A very healthy and popular choice of food for children. It is naturally high in protein and low in saturated fats and sodium. Chicken is also rich in selenium, which is essential for a healthy immune system. It also contains essential omega-3 and omega-6 fatty acids, niacin and vitamin B6.

Lamb

Lamb is a very good source of protein, iron, vitamin A, riboflavin, niacin, vitamin B12, zinc, copper and selenium. It also contains vitamin B6 pantothenic acid, phosphorous, and manganese. Vitamin

B12 and iron support the production of red blood cells while selenium has antioxidant properties, which help to boost the body's immune system while zinc is vital for brain function.

Pork

Pork is a great source of protein and iron and just like lamb and beef it also contains a whole range of vitamins and minerals, including potassium, selenium, zinc and magnesium, which are important for energy production and immune health. Pork also contains vitamin B6 and vitamin B12, which are vital for healthy brain function and tackling stress and anxiety

EGGS

A complete source of protein, they are rich in vitamin D, selenium, vitamin B12, iodine, iron and phosphorus. Eggs also contain the nutrient choline, which is used by the body to produce the neurotransmitter acetylcholine. Acetylcholine is involved in cognitive function and memory.

FRUITS

Apples

Apples are rich in the compound called pectin, which has been shown to reduce blood cholesterol levels and improve overall bowel health. Pectin helps carry cholesterol out of the digestive system. Apples also contain the plant compound called polyphenols, which have been shown to support immune health and lower inflammation in the body. Apples also contain high levels of a compound called quercetin, which has natural antihistamine activity. They are rich in vitamin C and fiber when eaten with the skin.

Bananas

Bananas are rich in dietary fiber, B vitamins and minerals especially potassium which is important for the functioning of the cells, nerves and muscles and can also relieve high blood pressure. Vitamins B5 and B6 help support the nervous system and combat the effects of stress. Their high starch content makes them a good source of sustained energy. Bananas are also rich in the amino acid tryptophan, which is known to lift the mood and aid sleep (body converts this amino acid into the 'feel good' neurotransmitter serotonin in the brain).

Blueberries

Blueberries are naturally high in antioxidant compounds called anthocyanidins, which give them their deep purple color and have been shown to protect blood vessel walls from damage and even reduce cholesterol slightly. They are also rich in vitamins C and E, selenium and zinc. Zinc is an essential mineral to help the brain turn glucose into energy as well as being needed for the production of hormones and neurotransmitters for brain function. Research has also shown that eating blueberries regularly can improve night vision. Blueberries are one of the wonderful superfoods for your child.

Cherries

Cherries are naturally rich in iron, potassium, vitamin C and B, as well as beta carotene. They contain high levels of compounds called anthocyanins, which gives them their deep ruby red color and has anti-inflammatory activity. They also contain a compound called melatonin, which helps to induce sleep. Cherries are also known to be a remedy for gout and arthritis in adults.

Dates

Dates are rich in dietary fiber, vitamin A, iron, potassium, calcium, manganese and copper. They are also packed with antioxidants known as tannins. Tannins are known to have anti-inflammatory and anti-hemorrhagic properties. Dates are high in sugars such as fructose and dextrose.

Figs

Figs are a well-known laxative and an excellent source of calcium and iron. They are rich in soluble fiber and natural sugars and are a good source of energy when energy levels are low.

Lemons

Lemons contain high levels of vitamin C, which is vital for immune function as it allows white blood cells to fight infection more ferociously. They also contain potassium, calcium, phosphorus, beta carotene and fiber. The membranes of the lemons contain bioflavonoids, which have powerful antioxidant properties.

Pears

Pears have large water content and are naturally high in vitamin C, fiber and potassium. They contain pectin and soluble fiber, which can help in lowering harmful cholesterol in the body. Pears are also rich in phytonutrients, which have antioxidant as well as anti-inflammatory benefits.

Peaches

Peaches are rich in vitamins C, E and K and antioxidants including carotenoids such as lycopene and lutein, which support the immune system and maintain healthy vision and skin. They are also a good source of potassium, which can help to maintain proper fluid balance and help regulate nerve and muscle activity.

Raspberries

Raspberries are rich in vitamin C and antioxidants, which help protect the body's cells and tissues against damage. They are also a good source of B vitamins including niacin and folate, which are important for the production of neurotransmitters, which support brain function. Raspberries are also rich in soluble fiber, which may help to keep blood sugar levels even through the day.

Strawberries

Strawberries are very rich in vitamin C – just three to four strawberries will provide a child with its daily requirement of this vitamin. They are also a good source of antioxidants such as anthocyanins, which may help to protect brain cells from damage. Strawberries also contain potassium and zinc, which helps to boosts mental function.

Papaya

Papaya are rich in vitamins A and C, folate, beta carotene, potassium and calcium. They also contain an enzyme called papain, which aids digestion and prevents bloating.

HERBS, SPICES AND SEASONINGS

Basil

Basil contains essential oils that relax the muscular walls of the small intestines and thus, have a calming effect on the stomach easing constipation, digestive cramps and bloating.

Cacao Powder

Cacao powder contains large amount of antioxidants called flavonoids, which keep high blood pressure down and reduce the blood's ability to clot. Cacao is rich in vitamins A, B1, B2, B3, C and pantothenic acid. It also contains a number of essential vitamins including magnesium, calcium, iron and potassium. Cocoa also helps to increase levels of the 'feel good' hormone serotonine in the brain. It also contains phenylethylamine, which acts as a slight antidepressant and stimulant similar to the body's own dopamine and adrenaline.

Cardamom

Cardamom is an aromatic spice that combats bloating and aids digestion. The essential oils of this spice help reduce gas and support natural rhythmic contractions of the gut.

Chilies

Chilies are rich in vitamin A, C, K, B6, potassium, copper and manganese. They also contain capsaicin – phytochemical that gives them their intense heat. Capsaicin causes the cells of our blood vessels to secrete nitric oxide, which helps the vessel walls to relax, so the vessels get wider and the circulation of blood improves to the extremities. Capsaicin also has painkilling effects.

Cilantro

Cilantro (coriander) is naturally rich in dietary fiber, vitamins, A, C, E, K, B6, calcium and iron. Cilantro is an effective digestive, easing indigestion and nausea.

Cinnamon

Cinnamon contains very good amounts of vitamin A, niacin, pantothenic acid, and pyridoxine. It has the highest antioxidant strength from all the food sources in nature. Cinnamon also contains an essential oil called eugenol, which has local anaesthetic and antiseptic properties.

Coconut Oil

This is one of the best oils to cook, it can be heated to high temperatures without being converted to trans fats. It is also an excellent energy booster, rich in medium chain triglycerides, which are converted via the liver into immediate energy rather than being stored by the body.

Cumin

Cumin is a very good source of vitamin B6, niacin, riboflavin, and other vital anti-oxidant vitamins like vitamins A, C, and E. The seeds are also rich in antioxidants, mainly carotene and lutein. Cumin aids digestion by increasing gut enzyme secretions.

Garlic

Garlic is rich in vitamin C, vitamin B6 and manganese. It has antimicrobial properties and is a natural antibiotic and when consumed help to protect you from bacterial, parasites and yeast infections. In addition, it also is known to have powerful anti-inflammatory properties, which may also protect against asthma. Garlic is also rich in sulphurous compounds that are responsible for liver detoxification and immune function.

Ginger

Ginger is naturally rich in vitamins B5 and B6, copper, potassium and magnesium. Potassium helps to control heart rate and blood pressure. Ginger has been in use since ancient times for its anti-inflammatory, carminative, anti-flatulent, and anti-microbial properties. It is also commonly used for treatment of nausea.

Honey
Honey is rich in antioxidants flavonoids, which help reduce the risk of some cancers and heart disease. It's made up of glucose, fructose and minerals such as calcium, iron, phosphate, potassium and magnesium. Honey is known for its anti-fungal and anti-inflammatory properties.

Lemon Grass
Lemon grass is rich in iron, potassium and manganese. The oils in lemon grass enhance blood circulation to extremities by relaxing the muscular walls of blood vessels, which, in turn, make them wider.

Olive Oil
Olive oil is very high in the omega-9 fatty acid called oleic acid, which helps to reduce levels of cholesterols. It also contains high levels of antioxidants called polyphenols, which help to reduce the blood clotting and also have anti-inflammatory properties.

Oregano
Oregano is a rich source of dietary fiber and minerals such as calcium, magnesium, potassium, copper and iron. It also contains beneficial essential oils called thymol, which have anti-bacterial and anti-fungal properties. Being naturally rich in vitamin A, carotenes and lutein, oregano is best known for its effective anti-oxidant properties.

Paprika
Paprika is rich in dietary fiber, vitamin A, vitamin C, vitamin E, vitamin K, riboflavin, niacin, iron and potassium. It's an excellent source of antioxidants carotenoids, specifically lutein and zeaxanthin that prevent harmful sunlight rays from damaging your eye tissues.

Parsley
Parley is an excellent source of vitamin C, iron and calcium. It also contains potent essential oils that help the kidney's filtration system by increasing the rate of fluid movement across the kidney filter, thereby increasing urinary output.

Peppercorns
Peppercorns are rich in dietary fiber, vitamin K, iron, copper and manganese. It's also believed to be a good remedy for constipation as it helps stimulate rhythmical contractions in the gut.

Rosemary

Rosemary is a good source of iron, calcium and vitamin B6. It is also naturally rich in antioxidants and anti-inflammatory compounds such as rosmarinic acid, which help boost the immune system and improve blood circulation. The essential oils in rosemary help widen the blood vessels, which in turn help to reduce blood pressure. Rosemary also contains an ingredient called carnosic acid that is able to fight off free radical damage in the brain.

Thyme

Thyme is rich in vitamin B6, A, C, E, K and folic acid. It is also a good source of potassium, iron, calcium and manganese. Thyme naturally contains an essential oil called thymol, which scientifically has been found to have antiseptic and anti-fungal characteristics.

Turmeric

Turmeric naturally contains high levels of vitamin C, B6, potassium, magnesium and manganese and is also a very good source of dietary fiber. Turmeric contains compounds called curcuminoids that have powerful anti-inflammatory properties and specifically, help protect the liver. These compounds help reduce inflammation and damage of liver cells (hepatocytes).

Vanilla

Vanilla extract is rich in B vitamins, which help in enzyme synthesis, nervous system function, and regulation of body metabolism. It also contains small traces of minerals such as calcium, potassium, zinc, iron and manganese. Vanilla contains the chemical called vanillin that may have cholesterol-lowering benefits.

RECIPES

Basic Recipes

•

Starters and Sharers

•

Soups and Salads

•

Mains

Meat

Seafood

Vegetarian

•

Desserts

BASIC RECIPES

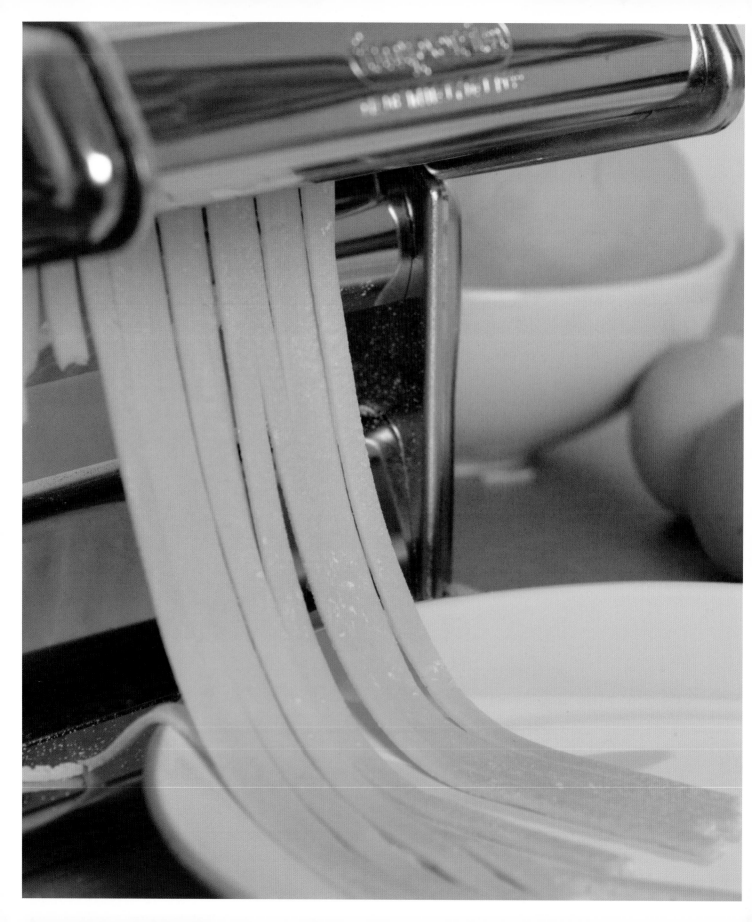

FRESH GLUTEN FREE PASTA

My children absolutely adore pasta. I don't know if this is something to do with their Italian genes or if it is simply due to all the different tastes, shapes and flavors that pasta comes in. Either way, pasta is such a versatile dish but when made fresh following this recipe, it really does make all the difference. The flavor and the texture of this pasta are excellent, highly palatable and perfectly even in consistency. As it is freshly made, it has a softer and more absorbent texture that easily takes on the flavors of the sauce with which it is served. I am thrilled that it is possible to make such a tasty and healthy gluten free pasta that is miles better than any dried gluten free pasta currently on the market. You can make a big batch of this fresh pasta and store it in the freezer for later use throughout the year. How convenient, how simple, how tasty!

400 g (14 oz) GF and DF bread flour mix (650 g white or brown rice flour, 250 g potato flour, 100g tapioca flour)
1 pinch salt
2½ tsp GF, DF, xanthan gum (only use if you are making your own bread flour mix)
4 eggs
3 tbsp extra virgin olive oil

1. To make fresh GF and DF pasta, use a good quality GF and DF flour mix – this can be found in all big supermarkets or from the internet. You can also make your own GF and DF flour mix by combining 650 g (1 lb 7 oz) of white or brown rice flour depending on your preference, 250 g (9 oz) of potato flour and 100 g (3.5 oz) of tapioca flour. This would make 1 kg (2.2lb) of GF and DF flour mix that you can store as normal flour.
2. Once you have your GF and DF flour mix ready, add the flour, a pinch of salt and xanthan gum into a bowl. Please only add xanthan gum if you are making your own flour mix as many other brands have already added the xanthan gum to their GF and DF flour mixes.
3. Break the eggs into a separate bowl and whisk lightly. Add the olive oil and whisk again.
4. Make a well in the center of the flour mixture, and pour in the egg and oil mix. Gently mix the mixture with a fork and bring together to make a stiff dough. Place the dough on a floured flat surface and knead for a few minutes until smooth.
5. Wrap dough tightly in cling film and allow to rest for at least 35 minutes.
6. Roll out using a pasta machine or by hand, and cut to the desired shape and length (tagliatelle, gnocchi, spaghetti etc)
7. Cook in boiling, salted water and serve with your favorite sauce or store in the freezer for later use.

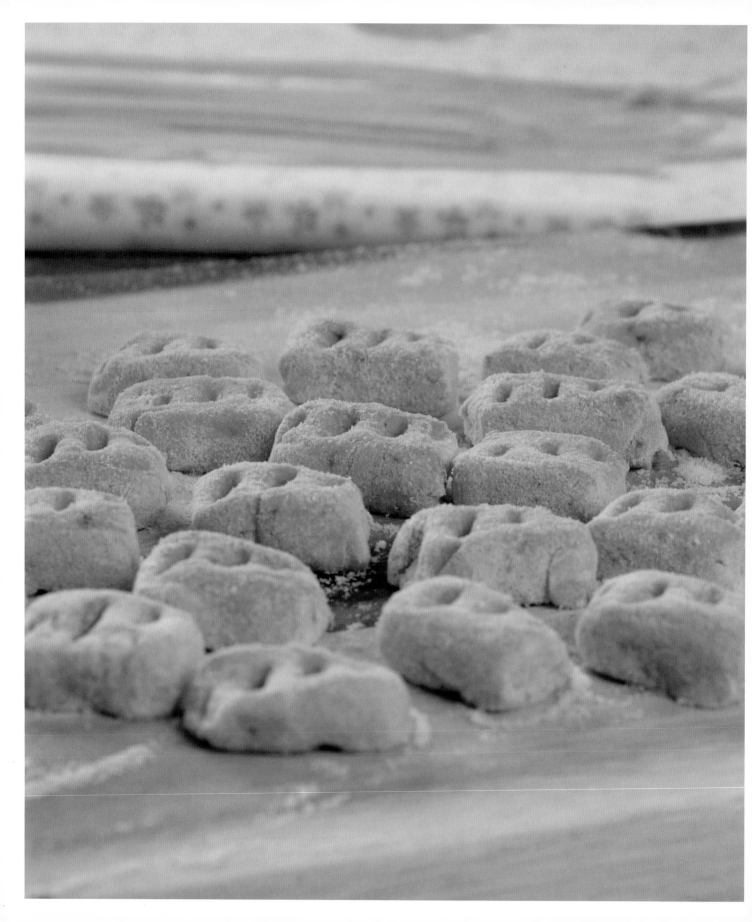

SWEET POTATOES AND BASIL GNOCCHI

These deliciously filling sweet potato dumplings are quick and easy to prepare. I like to use sweet potatoes due to its many nutritional and health benefits. In particular, they are rich in fiber, vitamin C, vitamin E, potassium and provide plenty of sustained energy. Sweet potatoes are also rich in antioxidants. Nowadays, you can easily buy ready-made gnocchi in the shops but always carefully read the ingredients section as most of the varieties are dusted with wheat flour.

Once cooked, serve with your favorite sauce.

400 g (14 oz) sweet potatoes
100 g (3.5 oz) white potatoes
2 egg yolks
125 g (4.5 oz) brown rice flour
2 tbsp fresh basil, finely chopped
salt to taste

1. Peel and cut the potatoes into large chunks and place them into a medium saucepan. Add cold water until the potatoes are covered by at least 2.5cm (1 inch) and bring it to the boil.
2. Cook for 15 minutes or until soft.
3. When the potatoes are done, drain the water, place them into a large bowl and let them cool down for 5 minutes. Mash the potatoes with a potato masher.
4. Add the egg yolks, brown rice flour, chopped basil, season with salt and mix well with your hands to form compact dough. Add more rice flour if the mixture is too sticky.
5. On a lightly floured surface, roll the dough into 30 cm (11 inches) long, 2 cm (¾ inch) wide cylinders. Keep the surface well-floured so that the gnocchi don't stick to it.
6. With a sharp knife, cut the cylinders into 3 cm (1¼ inch) long lengths and pattern them. Hold gnocchi against the prongs of the back of a fork, pressing only firmly enough to get the imprint of the fork.
7. Place them into a large floured container and refrigerate for 2 hours or freeze for later use.
8. To cook, boil gnocchi in salty water for 3–4 minutes or until they rise to the surface. Scoop them out with a slotted spoon and serve with your favorite sauce. (Best served with olive oil, salt and fresh thyme).

PERFECT GUACAMOLE

There are many different ways to make guacamole but this is the recipe that we love most in Casa Farina – indulgent, summery, fresh, rich and silky and nothing less than simply perfect guacamole. One constant ingredient in all guacamole recipes is a ripe avocado. Whenever possible, choose fresh and flavorful Hass avocados due to their extremely silky and buttery texture and mild and delicate flavor that perfectly blends with other ingredients. There are many guacamole recipes that call for a mayonnaise but I think you really do not need to, unnecessarily, add extra calories, ripe avocados are already very flavorful, creamy and rich. You can serve it either as a dip, condiment or with your favorite salad.

....

2 avocado, ripe and de-stoned
4 cherry tomato
1 handful of cilantro (coriander), finely chopped
1 shallot finely chopped
1 garlic clove, finely chopped
1 fresh red chili, deseeded and finely chopped
1 lime, juiced
salt

1. Place the tomatoes, cilantro, shallot, garlic and red chilies into a food processor and finely chop.
2. Scoop out the inner flesh of the avocado with a spoon, separating it from the outer skin. Place in a blender and add the lime juice and salt and blend 2 or 3 times in order not to over-process so that small chunks of avocado still remain in the mixture.
3. Add salt to taste and serve as a dip or as a side addition to a dish.

TOMATO SAUCE

A good tomato sauce is one of the first things you should learn to make before you attempt to do any cooking. There are countless uses of tomato sauce as well as countless ways of making it.

This basic four ingredient tomato sauce is a big success in Casa Farina and now it would be very difficult to imagine cooking without it, so, for the convenience, always make the sauce in batches and use in other dishes throughout the week.

....

2 tbsp virgin olive oil, for frying
1 large red onion, finely chopped
2 garlic cloves, crushed
1 handful fresh parsley, finely
  chopped
1 handful fresh basil finely chopped
2 tbsp tomato paste
60 ml (2 fl oz) water
1 liter (1 ¾ pint) tomato Passata
  (cooked and strained ripe
  tomatoes)
1 tsp brown sugar
2 carrots, peeled and cut in half
salt and pepper

1. Add two tablespoons of olive oil to a large size saucepan and gently fry the finely chopped onion for 5 minutes or until soft.
2. Add the garlic, parsley, basil and tomato paste, keep stirring for about 2 minutes. Then, add the water, tomato Passata, the salt, sugar and the carrots and simmer for a further 30 minutes or until the mixture thickens while still being liquid in consistency. Make sure you do not overcook it, as you still want to be able to pour rather than spoon your sauce. However, if you like your sauce thinner, add a splash of water.

* Tomato Passata is readily available in the supermarkets all over the World – this is the quickest way to obtain cooked and strained superior quality tomatoes.

PANGRATTATO

Pangrattato or 'poor people's Parmesan' as it was once called in Italy, has wonderful nutritional qualities, salty taste and works beautifully as a proxy for Parmesan. Use generously with your favorite pastas and baked dishes such as pies, lasagne, cannelloni or on salads, fish or chicken. A version of this Italian-inspired recipe has previously been used by poor people in Italy who couldn't afford to buy real Parmesan. I really like the taste of this Parmesan alternative, so much so that I now think it tastes even better than Parmesan. I like that, although very flavorful, it isn't at all heavy like Parmesan can be and it is a lot milder in taste too. It has fewer calories while also being rich in essential nutrients. Pangrattato beautifully accompanies a meal by adding that extra touch of crunchiness and flavor. So, there really is nothing not to like about this inexpensive yet incredibly delicious Parmesan substitute.

100 g (3.5 oz) GF breadcrumbs
3 tbsp fresh parsley, finely chopped
½ red chili, finely chopped
1 tbsp olive oil
salt and freshly ground black
pepper

1. Combine all the ingredients in a medium size bowl and gently mix.
2. In a non-stick frying pan, heat one tablespoon of olive oil on a medium heat, add the mixture and gently fry until completely dry and slightly browned.
3. Once cooked, let it cool and serve immediately as a Parmesan substitute or refrigerate for a few days in an airtight container for later use.

CREAMY BECHAMEL

Use this recipe as an alternative to cheese in baked dishes such as lasagne, cannelloni and some pies.

....

50 g (1.75 oz) corn flour (I like to use Maizena)
510 ml (18 fl oz) light coconut milk
25 g (1 oz) coconut oil
salt and pepper

1. In a medium size saucepan gently warm up the coconut milk.
2. In a bowl, place the corn flour (I like to use Maizena but any fine corn flour is good) and gently add the warm milk, whisking constantly.
3. Add the coconut oil, season with salt and pepper, mix well and pour the mixture back in the saucepan.
4. Cook the ingredients on a medium heat, stirring constantly until you obtain a smooth, thick, and creamy mixture.

HOMEMADE CHOCOLATE (GLUTEN, DAIRY, SOYA AND NUTS FREE)

This is a quick and easy chocolate recipe that is full of goodness and brilliant flavors. It's completely additives free too which, probably makes it to be one of the healthiest chocolates ever. You can use it as a dipping sauce or in baking some of your favorite chocolate desserts such as chocolate soufflé, (see page 190) or once well-set in a freezer, eat on its own as a usual chocolate treat. Raw cacao powder is rich in antioxidants, A, B and C vitamins, magnesium, iron, calcium and other nutrients and it also helps to increase levels of the 'feel good' hormone, serotonine, in the brain while it also acts as a mild antidepressant. On the other hand, coconut oil is completely cholesterol free and it doesn't contain any trans fatty acids either while xylitol is an ideal healthy sweetener which has 40% fewer calories than table sugar and a low glycaemic index which means it has a minimal impact on blood glucose levels unlike all other sugars. And to top it all off, xylitol has also been shown to help maintain healthy teeth. To smooth out the natural bitterness of the raw cacao powder and to get that vanilla aroma essence, always add a small amount (as indicated below) of vanilla bean paste. Enjoy!

60 g (2 oz) coconut oil
60 g (2 oz) date syrup
60 g (2 oz) raw cacao powder
½ tsp vanilla bean paste
25 ml (1 fl oz) coconut milk
a pinch of sea salt

1. Put the coconut oil, date syrup, raw cacao powder and vanilla bean paste into a medium size bowl and whisk well to combine all ingredients into a paste.
2. Pour in the coconut milk to obtain a silky texture.
3. Serve immediately as a dipping sauce or pour into chocolate moulds, freeze for 20 minutes and once the chocolate is set, gently pop the chocolate out of the moulds and serve.

TOP-NOTCH PANCAKES

A playful twist on the classic French crepe, this recipe is far lower in fat that traditional pancakes made with butter. For gluten, dairy and soya free version, always use gluten free flour and flavorful coconut milk. The possibilities for this easy to make and versatile dish are endless. Pancakes are an ideal base for cannelloni and lasagne as well as a perfect option for desserts and weekend breakfasts too. Serve rolled up or folded and filled with your favorite filling, sweet or sour.

180 g (6 oz) GF flour
3 eggs
150 ml (5 fl oz) coconut milk
350 ml (12 fl oz) water
1 tbsp fresh lemon juice
A pinch of salt
1 tbsp brown unrefined sugar
   (optional)

1. Place the flour into a large mixing bowl and make a well in the center. Crack the eggs into the middle, then pour about 100 ml of coconut milk and 150 ml of water, add one tablespoon of fresh lemon juice, one pinch of salt (and one tablespoon of sugar if you are making a batter for a pancake dessert).
2. Whisk from the center and slowly keep adding more water and milk until all the flour has been incorporated into the batter.
3. Whisk until you have a batter that is the consistency of a thin cream.
4. In the meantime, heat up a non-stick pancake pan over a high heat, then turn the heat down to medium to low. Wipe the pan with oiled kitchen paper and ladle some batter into it, tilting the pan to move the batter around for a thin and even layer.
5. Return the pan to the heat and leave to cook for 20–30 seconds or until golden brown underneath.
6. Carefully flip the pancake and cook for another 20–30 seconds. Stack on a plate and cover with another plate to keep warm while you make the rest.
7. Continue with the rest of the batter until you finish it.
8. Roll up and serve warm with your favorite filling: fruits, ice cream, chocolate or a whipped cream or use as a base to make lasagne or cannelloni.
9. Keep refrigerated for up to two days.

RASPBERRY AND GOJI BERRY COULIS

This irresistibly delicious and wonderfully fruity coulis is a perfect addition to your favorite desserts. Use generously on ice creams, custards, cakes or pour over your grilled fruits. The tangy and refreshing flavor of the raspberries blends perfectly well with the slightly sweet and sour flavor of goji berries. These fruits are rich in antioxidants, vitamins and minerals and are also well known for their many health benefits.

200 g (7 oz) fresh or frozen
   raspberries
60 g (2 oz) dried goji berries
2 tbsp fresh lemon juice
4 tbsp unrefined light brown sugar
   or xylitol

1. Put the dried goji berries into a small bowl, cover in warm water and soak for about 15 minutes or until very soft. Drain off and put aside.
2. Place the raspberries and soaked goji berries in a blender and blend until smooth.
3. Pass the mixture through a sieve into a bowl to separate the seeds from the juice.
4. Transfer the juice into a small pot, add lemon juice and sugar or xylitol and gently bring to the boil – reduce the heat to medium and keep stirring until the juice thickens and the mixture sticks to the spoon.
5. Leave it to cool and refrigerate for 30 minutes.
6. Generously pour over your favorite desserts and enjoy.
7. Keep the sauce refrigerated for up to a week.

DAIRY AND SOYA FREE WHIPPED CREAM

This is a playful twist on the classic shop bought whipped cream. As an excellent dairy and soya alternative, use cold coconut cream with a minimum of 28% of coconut milk fat.

This recipe is quick and easy as well as deliciously adaptable. Before you start whisking, you may also want to add a flavoring of your choice such as vanilla or orange extract, rum, cacao powder, fruit puree etc.

Once ready, use generously with your favorite desserts (e.g chocolate soufflé) or fruits. Nothing beats this irresistibly delicious, homemade, dairy and soya free whipped cream.

250 ml (8 fl oz) refrigerated coconut cream (28% or more of coconut milk fat)
4 tbsp light brown unrefined sugar or xylitol

1. Place the coconut cream into a fridge and refrigerate for a few hours until very cold.
2. Keep the cream refrigerated right up until you are ready to whip it so it is as cold as possible. On a very hot day, chill the bowl and the whisks before whisking.
3. Once the cream is cold, pour the cream into a stainless steel medium size bowl, add the sugar and whisk up. Before you start whipping, if you wish, you can add various flavorings to the mixture such as vanilla or orange extract, rum, cacao powder, fruit puree etc.
4. For whisking up, I like to use an electric hand mixer but you can also whisk it up manually or in a stand mixer with a whisk attachment.
5. Whisk on a medium setting for 4–5 minutes (if using an electric mixer) or until the cream starts taking on volume and the firm peaks form. Best time to stop whisking is when you remove the whisk out of the cream and the peaks in the whipped cream still hold firmly but have slightly softened tips. Make sure you do not whisk too long as you can break the fat apart and form a butter like consistency.
6. Once ready, serve immediately or cover with plastic wrap and store in the fridge for a few hours.

HORSERADISH MAYONNAISE

Nothing beats a rich and creamy homemade mayonnaise. It is so easy and quick to make yet tastes so delicious. Use it sparingly for dipping, as a base for other sauces or simply spread it on your wraps. In fact, just a touch of mayonnaise adds creamy goodness to all kinds of savory dishes.

As this recipe calls for raw egg yolk, make sure that you always use only fresh and refrigerated organic grade A eggs and also avoid the contact between the yolks and the shell.

Due to the slight risk of salmonella and other foodborne illnesses, this recipe is not recommended for pregnant women and small children.

1 egg yolk
1 tbsp white vinegar
1 tbsp fresh horseradish, grated
¼ tsp salt
200 ml (7 fl oz) light olive oil
1 tbsp fresh lemon juice
½ tsp Tabasco sauce

1. Place egg yolk, vinegar, grated horseradish and salt into a small bowl and whisk well.
2. Add the oil as slowly as you can to start with, whisking constantly until the oil is incorporated into the mixture and the sauce emulsifies and thickens. Do not use extra virgin olive oil as the flavor is too strong.
3. Whisk for up to 5 minutes or until you have a mixture that is the consistency of a thick and smooth cream.
4. At the end, add fresh lemon juice and Tabasco sauce, whisk well and serve or keep refrigerated for up to two days.

VANILLA CUSTARD SAUCE

This is a healthier alternative to traditional, calories laden vanilla custard.
It's perfect for slathering on puddings, crumbles and pies and is much
lighter than a traditional sauce as it does not contain any cream. OK, it
still won't make you lose weight and should really be used only sparingly
to add that extra smoothness and flavor to your favorite desserts.

450 ml (15 fl oz) coconut milk
1 tsp vanilla bean paste
4 egg yolks
50 g (1.5 oz) light brown
   granulated sugar
½ tsp corn flour
1 tbsp brandy/rum

Makes: 500 ml

1. In a medium size saucepan, bring the coconut milk and vanilla
paste to a boil over a low heat. Remove from the heat and let it to cool.
2. In a large bowl, cream the eggs and sugar. Add the corn flour and
mix well.
3. Slowly pour in the warm milk (not hot) whisking constantly until
all the milk has been incorporated.
4. Transfer the mixture back in the saucepan and cook over a low
heat, stirring constantly until the sauce thickens and coats the back
of the spoon.
5. Remove from the heat, add one teaspoon of brandy, mix well and
let it cool down quickly, placing the pan on top of cold water. Once
cool, cover with plastic wrap and refrigerate.
6. Serve with your favorite desserts.

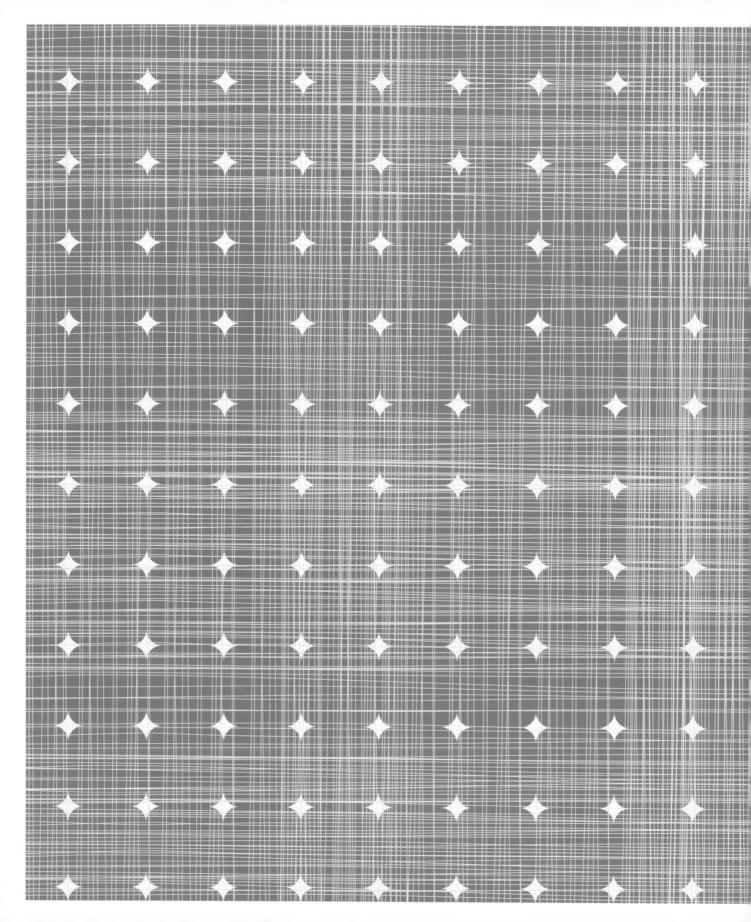

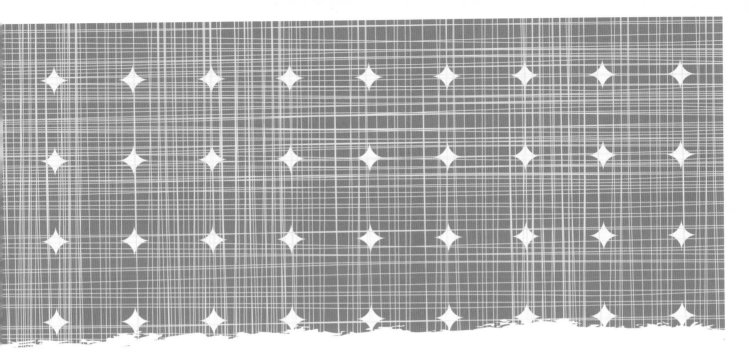

STARTERS AND SHARERS

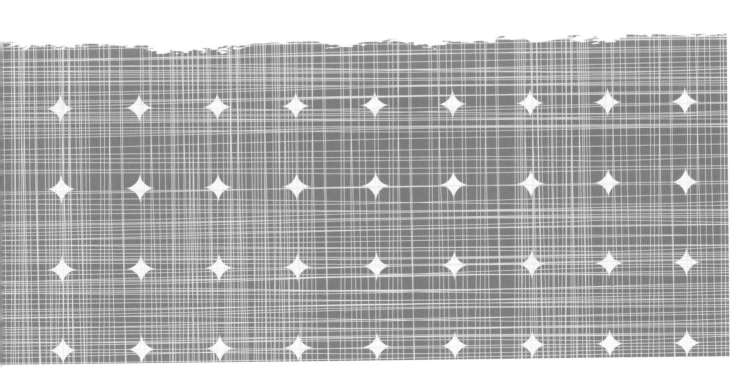

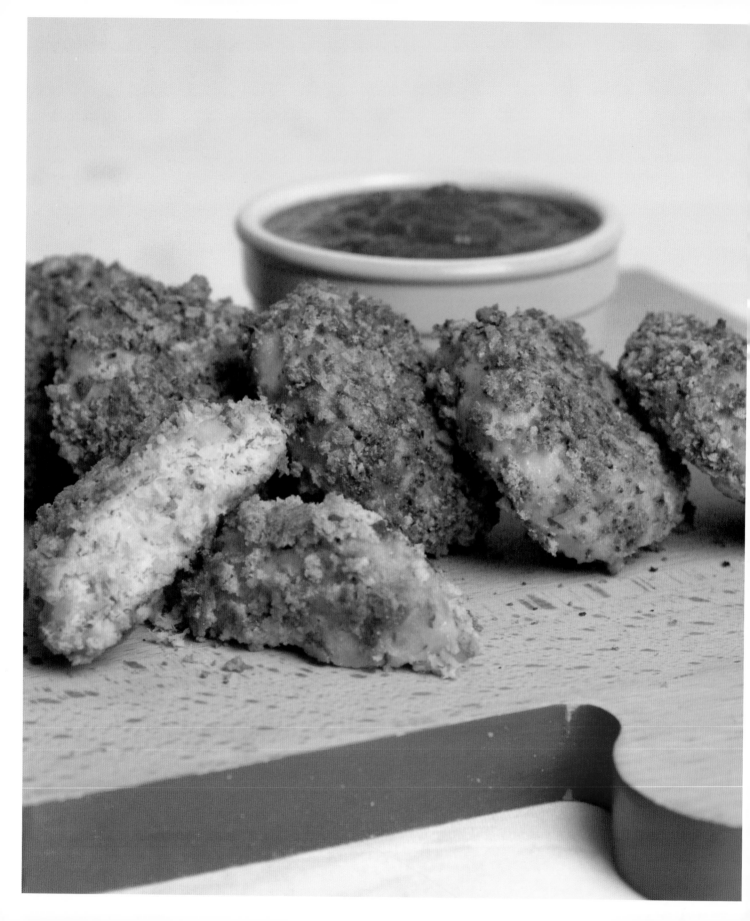

BAKED FISH CAKES

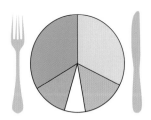

Rich and full of flavor, these little fish cakes are delicious hot or cold and make prefect nutritious starters or party sharers. And on the plus side, these cakes are baked rather than fried to reduce saturated fat content making them a healthy protein-packed option as an energy boosting snack. Fish is an excellent source of many vitamins and minerals, including vitamins A and D and selenium and is also rich in omega-3 fatty acids and proteins.

- ☐ Fruit & Vegetables
- ☐ Carbohydrates
- ☐ Milk, Dairy or Alternatives
- ☐ High in Sugar and/or Fat
- ☐ Proteins

300 g (10.5 oz) salmon fillet
100 g (3.5 oz) cod fillet
60 g (2 oz) smoked mackerel (boneless)
300 g (10.5 oz) white potatoes
250 ml (8 fl oz) coconut milk
1 handful of fresh parsley, finely chopped
1 tbsp lemon juice (fresh)
2 scallions (spring onions)
1 tbsp ketchup
2 tbsp fresh chives, finely chopped
2 eggs, beaten
100 g (3.5 oz) GF wholemeal breadcrumbs
salt and freshly ground black pepper to taste

Serves: 4
Preparation Time: 20 min
Cooking Time: 30 min

1. Preheat the oven to 190°C (375°F).
2. Boil potatoes until soft, drain and put into a large bowl.
3. In the meantime, place the fish in a shallow pan (with a lid) and add just enough coconut milk until the fish is half covered. Heat until the milk is just beginning to boil, turn the heat down, cover, and let simmer for about 5 minutes or until fish is cooked well in the center and flakes easily. Drain the fish thoroughly, skin it (if necessary) and flake it, removing any bones.
4. Mash the potatoes, stir in the flaked fish and add smoked mackerel, chopped parsley, lemon juice, chopped scallions, ketchup, chopped chives and one beaten egg. Season with salt and pepper and mix thoroughly.
5. Shape the mixture into small patties and coat in the beaten egg and breadcrumbs (firstly, dip the cakes into a beaten egg, then coat it with the GF breadcrumbs for extra crunchiness).
6. Place into the baking tray onto a non-stick paper, spray the olive oil over the fish cakes and bake for 30 minutes until crisp and golden.
7. Serve warm or cold.

SALMON SKEWERS WITH POMEGRANATE AND BALSAMIC VINEGAR GLAZE

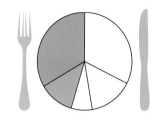

- ■ Fruit & Vegetables
- □ Carbohydrates
- □ Milk, Dairy or Alternatives
- □ High in Sugar and/or Fat
- ■ Proteins

This is one of the well-known old favorites with a little twist – pomegranate and balsamic vinegar glaze instead of a very commonly used soya derived glaze. The combination of pomegranate and vinegar glaze works just heavenly together making this dish one of my all time favorites. And above everything, it's healthy too: packed with omega-3 fatty acids, proteins, insoluble fiber, B and many other vitamins while still being low in fat. My whole family loves this easy to make nutritious and highly flavorsome recipe. Kids just can't wait to get their skewers on the plate so they can start competing over who will be first to take off all the fish and vegetables.

....

260 g (9 oz) salmon fillet (2 fillets)
2 cherry tomatoes
½ zucchini (courgette)
½ yellow pepper
1 tbsp balsamic vinegar
2 tbsp pomegranate molasses
1 tbsp wild honey

Serves: 4
Preparation Time: 10 min
Cooking Time: 10 min

1. Preheat the grill to high.
2. Cut the salmon fillets and vegetables into cubes.
3. In a separate small bowl, mix well the balsamic vinegar, pomegranate molasses and honey together to create a glaze.
4. Take a skewer (metal or wooden) and thread alternating cubes of salmon and vegetables onto it.
5. Brush the glaze lightly over the skewers, place them under the grill and grill for about 10 minutes, turning occasionally.
6. Serve warm.

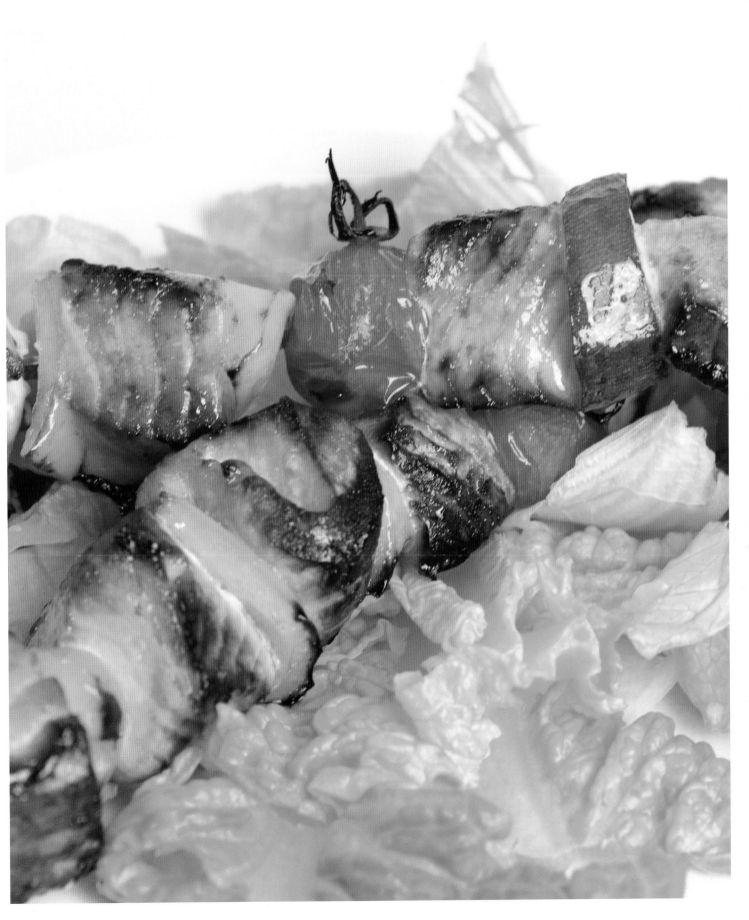

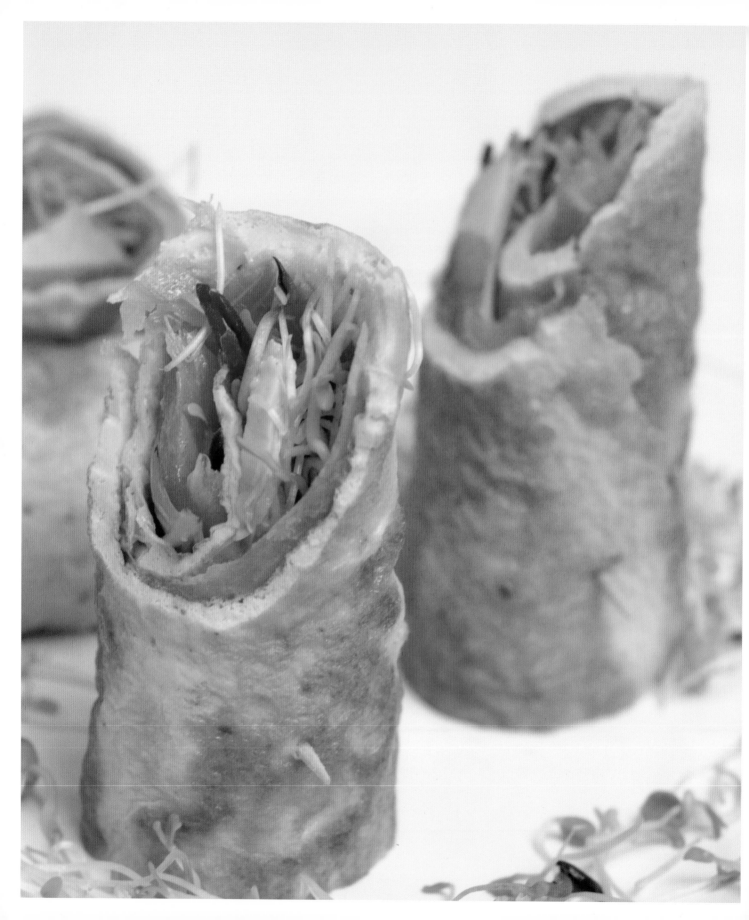

OMELETTE ROLLS WITH SMOKED SALMON

- ■ Fruit & Vegetables
- □ Carbohydrates
- □ Milk, Dairy or Alternatives
- □ High in Sugar and/or Fat
- ■ Proteins

This delicious 'grab and go' dish makes an elegant starter or a party sharer. It's made in minutes and yet is so tasty and nutritious. Smoked salmon is an excellent source of omega-3 fatty acids, energizing B vitamins and selenium while eggs are a complete source of proteins and are rich in vitamin D, vitamin B12 and phosphorus. To fill the rolls, use a selection of fresh vegetables of your choice. Vegetables are a good source of many antioxidants, dietary fiber, essential vitamins and minerals.

After trying these flavorful omelette rolls, scrambled eggs on toast will become a thing of the past.

....

3 eggs
1 tbsp olive oil
150 g (5 oz) smoked salmon
1 handful of fresh basil leaves
1 carrot, julienne
½ ripe avocado, sliced
1 fresh beetroot, finely sliced
20 g (¾ oz) alfalfa and radish
  shoots mix (optional)
Salt to taste
2 tsp mayonnaise

Serves: 2
Preparation Time: 10 min
Cooking Time: 5 min

1. Crack the eggs and place into a medium size bowl. Season with salt and whisk well.
2. In the meantime, heat the olive oil in a non-stick frying pan (medium size, 20-cm/8-inch) on a medium heat. Carefully, ladle half of the egg mixture into the pan. Tilt to coat the bottom of the pan and cook for 2 minutes or until set, carefully flip over and cook on the other side.
3. Make a second omelette wrap in the same way.
4. Spread mayonnaise in a thin layer over each omelette wrap, place smoked salmon slices and a selection of finely cut vegetables into the center and roll up tightly. In this recipe, I used avocado, carrot, beetroot, basil leaves and alfalfa and radish shoots mix, although you can use a selection of any fresh vegetables that like to eat.
5. Cut each wrap in half and then cut each piece diagonally in half again and secure the rolls with cocktail sticks.
6. Serve warm or cold.

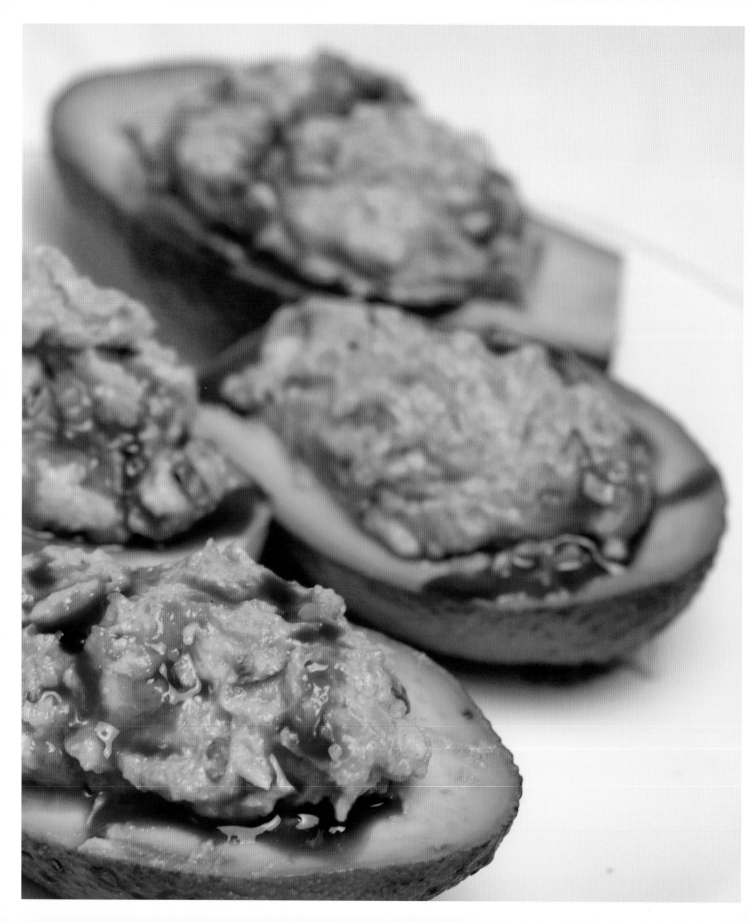

SHRIMP AND CRAB DRESSED AVOCADO

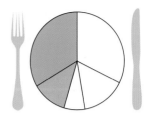

- ■ Fruit & Vegetables
- □ Carbohydrates
- □ Milk, Dairy or Alternatives
- □ High in Sugar and/or Fat
- ■ Proteins

This easy to make and irresistibly delicious appetizer is full of nutrients and flavor. Crab is packed with omega-3 fats and easily digestible proteins, shrimps are rich in antioxidants and immune supporting minerals such as zinc and selenium while avocado is a good source of energizing B vitamins and monosaturated fats. Evocative and delicate, the sweet holiday taste of crab and shrimps blends perfectly with the fresh, creamy and satisfying texture of avocados. This recipe calls for brown crabmeat because of its stronger sea-like taste but you can also use white crabmeat instead or a mix of both, white and brown meats. This recipe is an easy appetizer solution when you have little time to cook but you still want to impress your guests.

....

200 g (7 oz) cooked small shrimp (prawns)
100 g (3.5 oz) cooked brown crab meat
2 tbsp mayonnaise
1 tbsp tomato ketchup (optional)
1 tbsp basil, finely chopped
5 drops Tabasco sauce
2 avocados, halved and de-stoned
Salt and freshly ground black pepper to taste
Balsamic vinegar glaze to decorate

Serves: 4
Preparation Time: 10 min +
30 min chilling
Cooking Time: N/A

1. Add the shrimp, brown crab meat, mayonnaise, tomato ketchup (optional), finely chopped basil, 4–5 drops of Tabasco in a medium size bowl. Season with salt and pepper and mix well.
2. Cut an avocado in half and de-stone – hold the fruit in both hands and twist the two halves apart. Gently roll the stone out or carefully use the middle of a knife blade to gently stab the stone to twist it out.
3. Spoon the shrimp and crab mixture into avocado halves, piling quite high.
4. Place in the fridge and chill for 30 minutes. (If all the ingredients have already been in the fridge prior to preparation, serve the dish straightaway).
5. After chilling, garnish with balsamic vinegar glaze and serve.

BAKED EGGPLANT AND OLIVE PATTIES

These irresistibly delicious patties are full of summery Mediterranean flavors and essential nutrients. Eggplants are a good source of antioxidants and soluble fiber while green olives are rich in iron and vitamin E. Olives blend beautifully with the flesh of the eggplant to make wonderfully moist patties that are loved by everyone.

800 g (1 lb 12 oz) eggplants
   (aubergines) (2–3 medium size)
1 tbsp olive oil
1 large egg
80 g (3 oz) GF breadcrumbs
60 g (2 oz) green olives, finely
   chopped
1 garlic clove, crushed
1 handful of parsley, finely chopped
50 g (1.75 oz) corn meal
salt and freshly ground black pepper
   to taste

Serves: 4
Preparation Time: 10 min
Cooking Time: 60 min

1. Preheat oven to 200°C (400°F).
2. Cut eggplant lengthways in halves, carefully cut through the flesh down to the skin, taking care not to cut through the skin. Place them side by side on a baking tray, drizzle with olive oil, season with salt and bake for 45 minutes or until the flesh is soft and slightly browned.
3. Remove the eggplants from the oven, let them cool and carefully scoop the flesh out of the baked eggplant halves, place into a strainer and press down to remove all the excess water. Put the flesh on a clean chopping board and finely chop.
4. Place the eggplants into a medium size bowl, add egg, GF breadcrumbs, finely chopped olives, garlic, parsley and season with salt and pepper (adjust the quantity of salt depending on how salty the green olives are).
5. Mix well to form moderately stiff dough.
6. Take one tablespoon of the mixture and shape with your hands into a small patty. Repeat until you have used all the mixture.
7. Add the corn maize into a deep plate, gently coat the patties with the corn on all sides, place onto a non-stick parchment paper lined baking tray and bake for 15 minutes or until golden brown.
8. Serve warm or cold with your favorite dip or with crunchy salad.

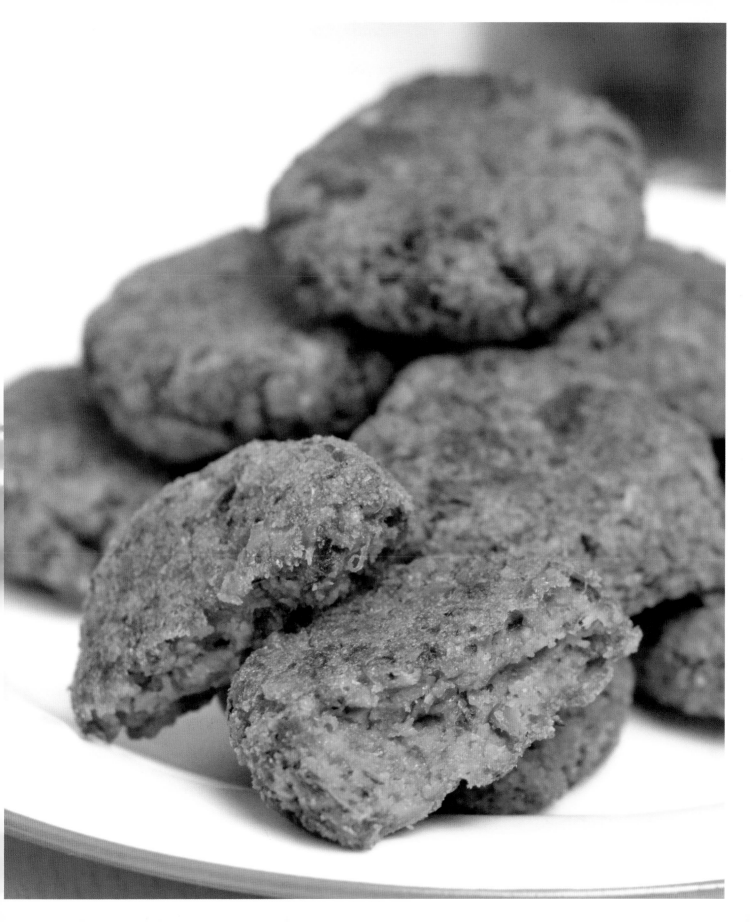

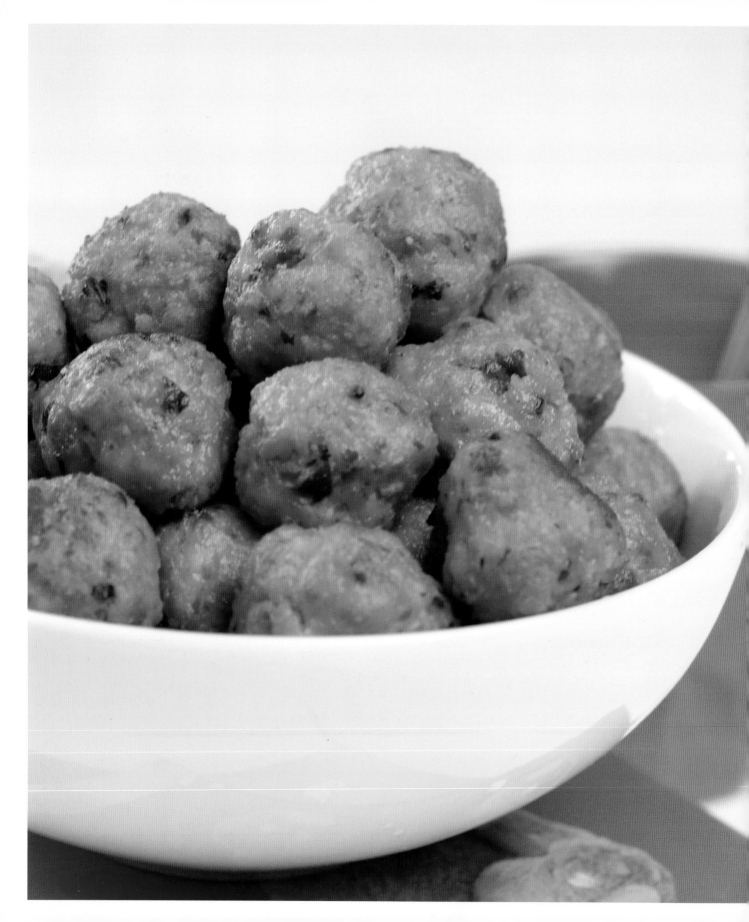

TURKEY MEATBALLS

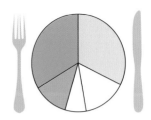

This delicious, 'grab & go' dish is very popular in Casa Farina, especially when the little friends are around. The meatballs are packed with nutrients, good for sharing, and help to satisfy even the hungriest of guests. Apart from being a perfect dish for parties, it's also an excellent choice for children's lunch boxes. When meatballs are around, nobody ever leaves hungry!

- ☐ Fruit & Vegetables
- ☐ Carbohydrates
- ☐ Milk, Dairy or Alternatives
- ☐ High in Sugar and/or Fat
- ☐ Proteins

....

250 g (9 oz) minced turkey (thigh)
1 handful of fresh parsley, finely chopped
1 handful of fresh basil, finely chopped
1 apple grated
1 egg
70 g (2.5 oz) GF wholemeal breadcrumbs
1 tbsp corn flour
1 tbsp lemon juice (fresh)
1 tsp paprika (sweet)
A pinch of salt
A pinch of raw cane sugar or xylitol
Coconut oil, for frying

Serves: 4
Preparation Time: 15 min + 30 min resting
Cooking Time: 30 min

1. In a large bowl combine the minced turkey, finely chopped parsley and basil, grated apple, egg, breadcrumbs, corn flour, lemon juice, paprika and season with salt and sugar.
2. Mix all the ingredients well (best done with your hands) until you get a firm mixture.
3. Cover the bowl with cling film and refrigerate for 30 minutes. This will help meatballs to firm and will stop them from falling apart.
4. After 30 minutes, roll the mixture out and shape into 3 cm (1¼ inch) large balls.
5. Heat the coconut oil in a medium frying pan over a high heat (pour 2 cm (¾ inch) of oil in a pan, ensuring that the meatballs are half way covered).
6. Ensure that the oil is very hot when you drop the meatballs into it – hot oil will quickly seal the outer edges of the meatballs minimizing the amount of oil that seeps into the meatballs while you will still get all the crispiness and flavor.
7. Carefully transfer the meatballs into the oil and fry, (turning occasionally) until golden brown on all sides.
8. Leave to cool for 5–10 minutes before serving.

67

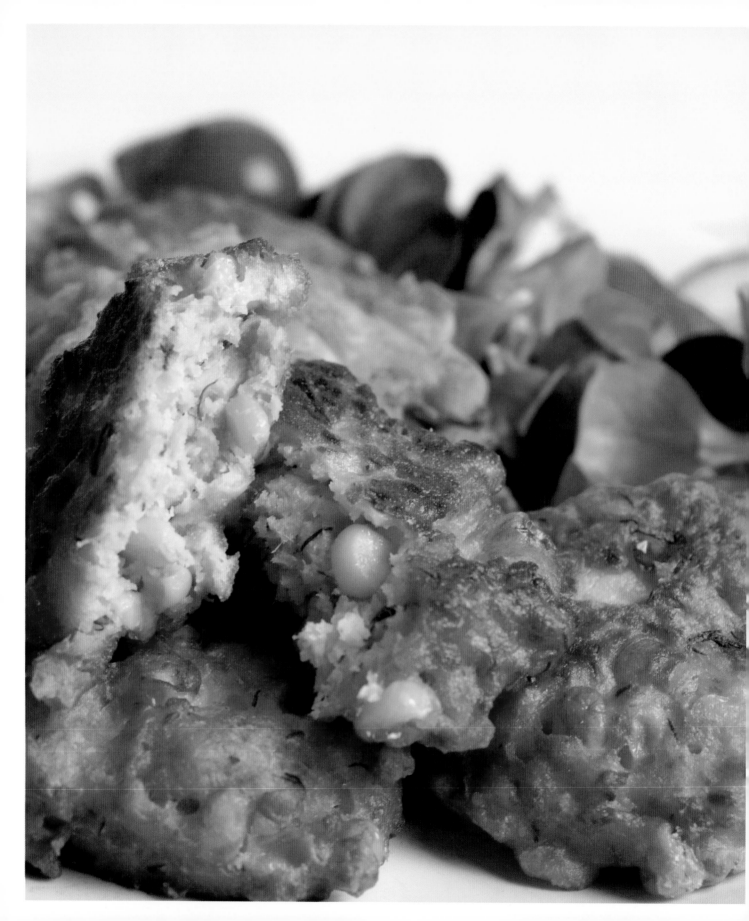

TUNA, SALMON AND CORN FRITTERS

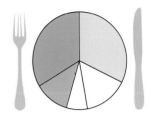

Made in minutes, wonderfully tasty and packed with nutrients – these fritters are an ideal solution when you really don't know what to cook but want to prepare something easy, quick and nutritious, and above all, something that your little ones would love too. You can have these as an appetizer or as a main course with a crunchy salad on the side. Tuna and salmon will provide you with plenty of protein, iron and good omega-3 fats while sweet corn is packed with energizing B and C vitamins, manganese and magnesium. My kids love to say they are eating burgers rather than fritters as in their eyes, anything that looks like a burger, must be a burger. I don't complain at all knowing that they get even more good nutrients eating these so everyone is happy in the end.

☐ Fruit & Vegetables
☐ Carbohydrates
☐ Milk, Dairy or Alternatives
☐ High in Sugar and/or Fat
☐ Proteins

2 tbsp olive oil
3 garlic cloves, finely chopped
1 red onion, finely chopped
200 g (7 oz) salmon fillet, cut into
    small pieces
400 g (14 oz) frozen corn kernels
3 eggs
120 g (4 oz) canned tuna chunks in
    olive oil, drained
30 g (1 oz) GF flour
30 g (1 oz) corn flour
1 tbsp fresh dill, finely chopped
Sea salt and freshly ground black
    pepper

Makes: 20 fritters
Preparation Time: 10 min
Cooking Time: 10 min

1. Heat the olive oil in a large non-stick pan. Add the chopped garlic and onion and gently fry, stirring occasionally, until soft and golden brown.
2. Add the salmon and the frozen corn kernels, mix well and cook for a further 5 minutes.
3. Place the fried mixture in a large bowl and add the eggs, tuna, GF flour, corn flour and the chopped dill. Season with salt and freshly ground black pepper and mix thoroughly to combine all the ingredients.
4. In a separate large non-stick frying pan, add olive oil and heat over a medium heat. Spoon tablespoons of the fish and corn mixture into the pan and repeat until you fill the pan.
5. Cook for about 2 minutes on each side or until the fritters are golden brown and well cooked in the middle.
6. Once cooked, remove the fritters and drain them on absorbent paper before serving.
7. Serve warm or cold.

CALAMARI FRITTI

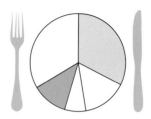

☐ Fruit & Vegetables
☐ Carbohydrates
☐ Milk, Dairy or Alternatives
☐ High in Sugar and/or Fat
▣ Proteins

This is a delicious, easy and healthier version of the classic recipe, which however, requires three essential criteria to get it right: fresh squid, for the taste, dried well, for the lightness and hot frying oil, for the crispiness. It is really important that the frying oil is very hot, if the oil is hot enough, when the squid is dropped in it, the outer edges of the squid quickly seal, minimizing the amount of oil that will seep into the squid while you still get all the crispiness and flavor. The recipe usually calls for a plain flour but here I am using a corn flour for that extra crispiness and better taste. Squids are a good source of protein, low in fat and sodium and rich in B12 vitamin, which is important for red blood cell production, nervous system health and niacin which is important for metabolism. This dish is a winner every time and you will, most definitely, have your guests asking for more.

1 liter (1 ¾ pint) light frying oil
500 g (1 lb 2 oz) medium size fresh squids, (cleaned and sliced)
60 g (2 oz) corn flour
1 fresh lemon, halved (optional)
salt and freshly ground black pepper

Serves: 4
Preparation Time: 15 min
Cooking Time: 10 min

1. Fill a large, heavy based frying pan a third full with a good quality olive oil for frying and heat over medium-high heat until a pinch of flour sizzles when it hits the oil.
2. Remove the skin of the squid (or get your fishmonger to do it) and wash the squid tubes well in a cold water
3. Slice the tubes into approximately 7mm rings. Drain excess water and dry them well with an absorbent kitchen paper.
4. Place the corn flour, salt and pepper into a freezer bag, mix well and then place the squid rings into the bag. Close the bag, shake well and ensure the rings are well coated with the corn flour on all sides.
5. Remove the squid rings from the bag, handful by handful. Shake off the excess flour and place them gently into the hot oil.
6. Fry in batches for 2–3 minutes until crisp and golden brown.
7. Place on kitchen paper, sprinkle with salt, and serve immediately. Best served with lemon wedges and/or mayonnaise.

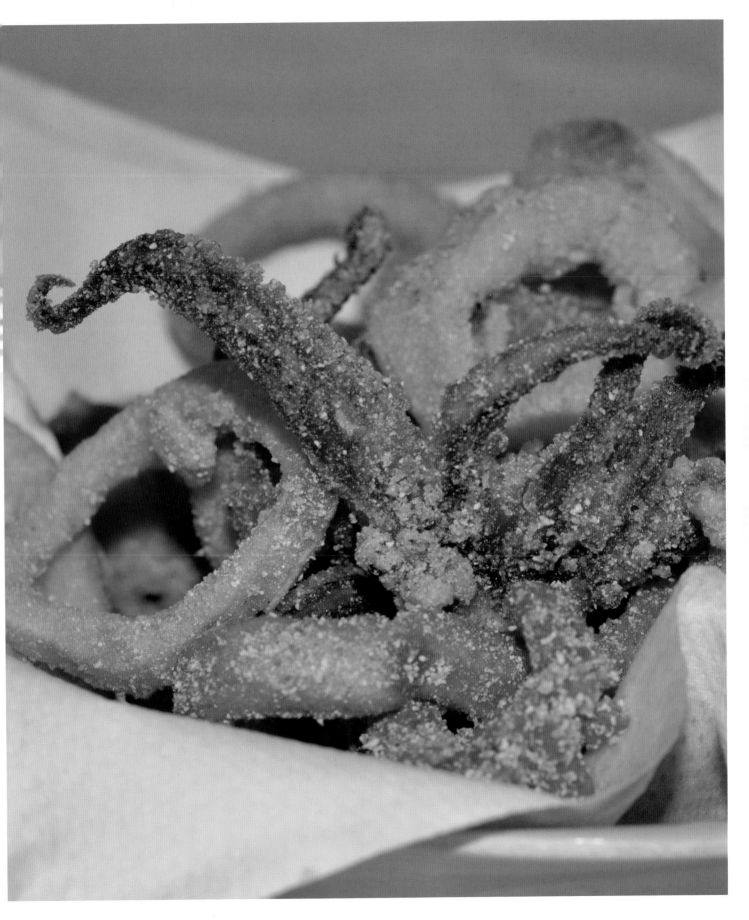

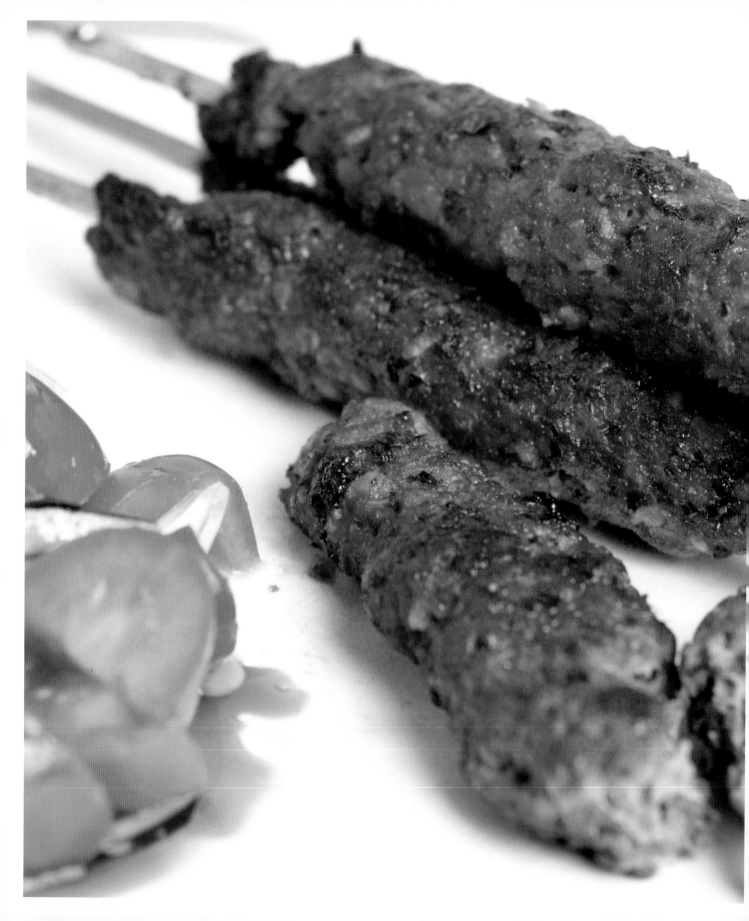

GRILLED LAMB KOFTAS

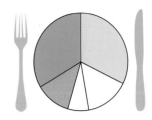

This is a healthy energy booster, packed with proteins and iron. Ideal for toddlers who are always on the go, like my children, but it is also good for parties or as a protein-packed starter. Apple blends beautifully with lamb mince to make wonderfully moist and tasty koftas and having them grilled rather than fried, makes all the difference. Grilling results in a minimal loss of moisture and vitamins, significantly reduces the fat content and the food also retains more of a nutritional content.

■ Fruit & Vegetables
☐ Carbohydrates
☐ Milk, Dairy or Alternatives
☐ High in Sugar and/or Fat
■ Proteins

500 g (1 lb 2 oz) minced lamb
1 red onion
1 handful of fresh parsley
1 handful of fresh basil leaves
1 garlic clove, crushed
1 apple, grated and drained
2 tbsp olive oil
1 tbsp grated fresh ginger
1 tbsp tomato paste
1 tsp ground cumin
1 tbsp paprika
1 tsp dry oregano
2 tsp ground cilantro (coriander)
1 tsp cayenne pepper
1 tbsp GF flour
Salt
6 skewers

Serves: 4
Preparation Time: 15 min + 30 min resting
Cooking Time: 12 min

1. Preheat grill (medium heat) or barbecue.
2. Finely chop the onion, parsley, basil and garlic, (best done using a mini electric chopper).
3. In a large bowl, mix minced lamb with chopped onion, garlic, grated apple, GF flour and basil. Add olive oil, ginger and tomato paste.
4. Season with salt, cumin, paprika, oregano, cilantro and cayenne pepper and mix well.
5. Cover with plastic wrap and leave in the fridge to chill for 30 minutes.
6. Divide the mixture to 6 even portions and shape each portion into a sausage like shape around the skewers.
7. Place the skewers horizontally on the edges of the baking tray ensuring that only the skewers and not the meat are touching the tray. This method of cooking will significantly reduce fat content of the koftas (fat drips off as the meat cooks).
8. Grill for 10–12 minutes on medium heat or until well done, rotating every 3–4 minutes until golden brown.
9. Serve immediately.

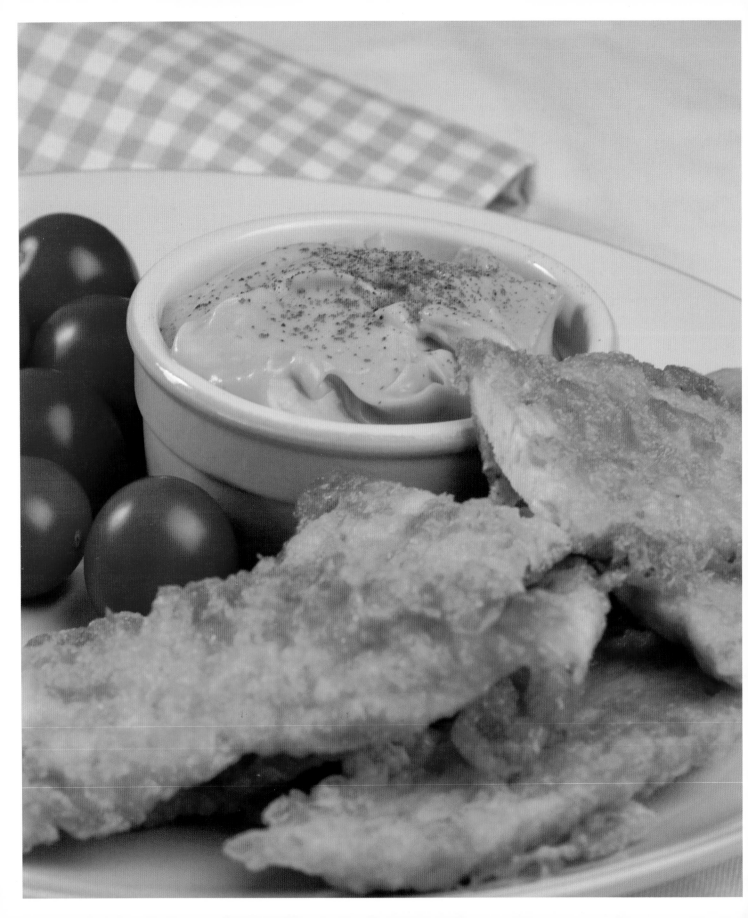

MINI CHICKEN MILANESE

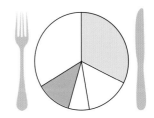

This beautifully golden and crispy mini chicken Milanese is an excellent energy booster for your active little ones. It's super easy to make and is packed with tons of flavor. It can be eaten on its own as a 'grab & go' snack, as a sharer at parties or accompanied with spaghetti as a main course; the possibilities for this versatile dish are endless. Children as well as adults simply love it.

☐ Fruit & Vegetables
☐ Carbohydrates
☐ Milk, Dairy or Alternatives
☐ High in Sugar and/or Fat
▣ Proteins

300 g (10.5 oz) mini organic chicken fillets
4 tbsp fine corn meal
2 tbsp corn flour
A pinch of salt
A pinch of paprika
2 eggs
4 tbsp coconut oil for frying

Dip
4 tbsp DF and GF mayonnaise
2 tbsp ketchup
½ tsp smoked paprika
A pinch of salt
3 cm (1¼ in) cucumber, finely grated

Serves: 4–6
Preparation Time: 15 min
Cooking Time: 10 min

1. For the Chicken Milanese: place the mini chicken fillets on a chopping board and gently beat with a meat mallet until flat (no more than 5–7mm in thickness).
2. In a large bowl mix corn meal, corn flour, salt and paprika.
3. In a separate bowl, beat the eggs.
4. Heat coconut oil in a large skillet over medium heat.
5. Gently coat the fillets in the flour mixture, working with one piece at a time.
6. Once the oil gets hot, dip the coated fillets into the beaten eggs and gently fry until crisp and golden brown (approximately 4 minutes on each side).
7. Place the chicken on absorbent kitchen paper allowing the excess oil to drain.
8. Serve warm or cold with or without a dip.
9. For the Dip: place DF and GF mayonnaise, ketchup, paprika, salt and cucumber in a bowl and mix thoroughly.
10. Spoon the dip into a separate small side bowl and serve with Chicken Milanese.

SOUPS AND SALADS

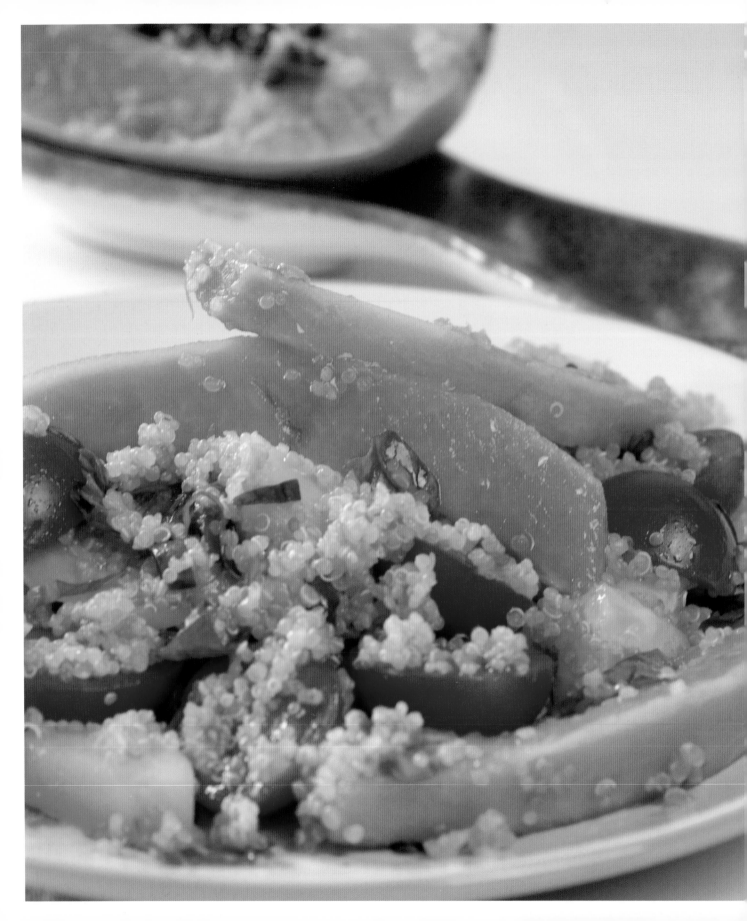

SUPER HEALTHY QUINOA AND ANCHOVY SALAD

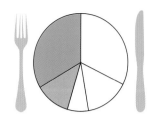

- ■ Fruit & Vegetables
- ☐ Carbohydrates
- ☐ Milk, Dairy or Alternatives
- ☐ High in Sugar and/or Fat
- ■ Proteins

This salad combines delicious flavors of summer with papaya, cherry tomatoes, cucumbers and protein-rich quinoa. The flavors are heightened with the anchovy vinaigrette for a healthy twist and near-gourmet experience. Its vibrant color is sure to catch your children's attention and they will love the delicious, exotic, sweet and salty combination of flavors. After all, not all salads are green and boring.

Salad

100 g (3.5 oz) quinoa
6 cherry tomatoes, cut in half
½ cucumber, diced
1 avocado, diced
1 papaya, sliced

Anchovy Vinaigrette

1 tbsp olive oil
½ anchovy paste
½ lemon (for lemon juice)
½ tsp sweet balsamic vinegar

Serves: 4
Preparation Time: 10 min
Cooking Time: 10 min

1. For the Salad: first, rinse the quinoa in the water to remove its bitter coating.
2. Add the quinoa into a pan of water, (two cups of water to one cup of grain) cover, bring to boil, simmer and cook for around 15 minutes or until the germ separates from the seed. Leave to cool.
3. Add sliced cherry tomatoes, cucumber, avocado and papaya into a large bowl, stir in the fluffy quinoa and gently mix.
4. Season and serve immediately.
5. For the Anchovy Vinaigrette: in a small bowl add olive oil, anchovy paste, a good squeeze of fresh lemon juice and half teaspoon of balsamic vinegar. Mix gently.
6. Drizzle over the salad and serve.

QUINOA AND SPINACH SALAD WITH POMEGRANATE GLAZE

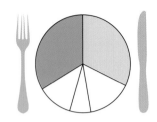

- ◼ Fruit & Vegetables
- ◻ Carbohydrates
- ◻ Milk, Dairy or Alternatives
- ◻ High in Sugar and/or Fat
- ◻ Proteins

This delightful and easy to make salad offers all the nutritious benefits of protein- and fiber-rich quinoa, iron-rich spinach, B vitamins and monosaturated fats-rich avocado and antioxidants rich pomegranate. It's a perfect colorful summer dish on its own or as a side with fish or chicken.

....

100 g (3.5 oz) quinoa
150 ml (5 fl oz) vegetable stock
30 g (2 oz) baby spinach
1 avocado, sliced
1 pomegranate (fresh)
2 tbsp pomegranate molasses
1 pinch of salt (optional)

Serves: 2
Preparation Time: 10 min
Cooking Time: 10 min

1. Rinse the quinoa in cold water in a fine-mesh strainer.
2. Bring the vegetable stock to a boil and stir in the quinoa.
3. Uncover and simmer for about 10 minutes or until a small spiral becomes visible in each grain. Drain the quinoa and transfer it to a medium bowl.
4. Add the spinach and toss with the hot quinoa until slightly wilted. Add the sliced avocado and toss again.
5. Generously sprinkle the salad with the fresh pomegranate seeds and glaze with 2 tablespoons of the pomegranate molasses.
6. Serve immediately.

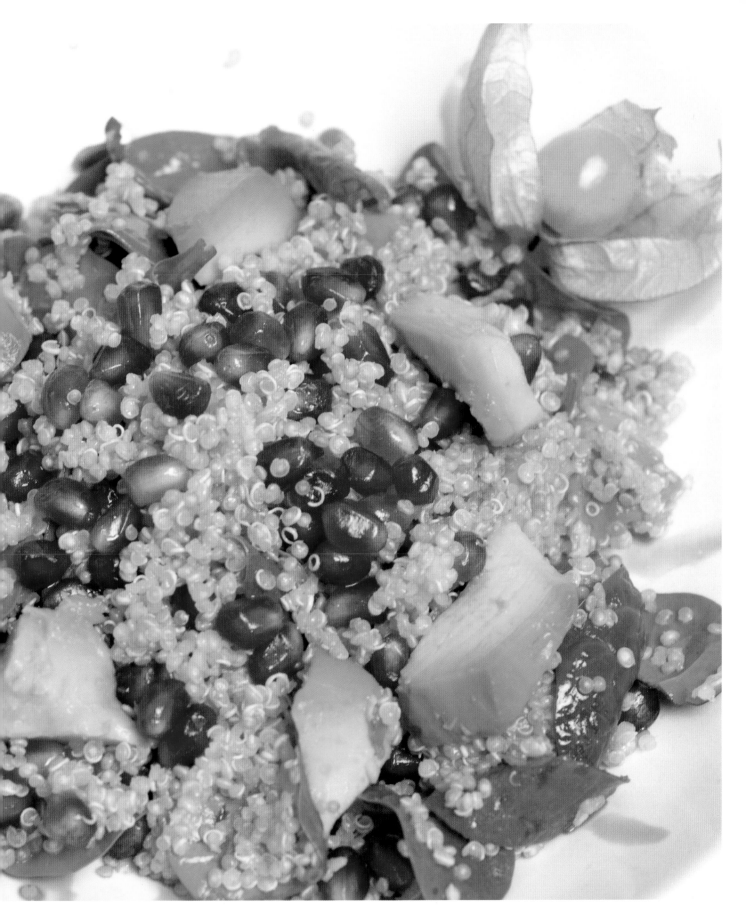

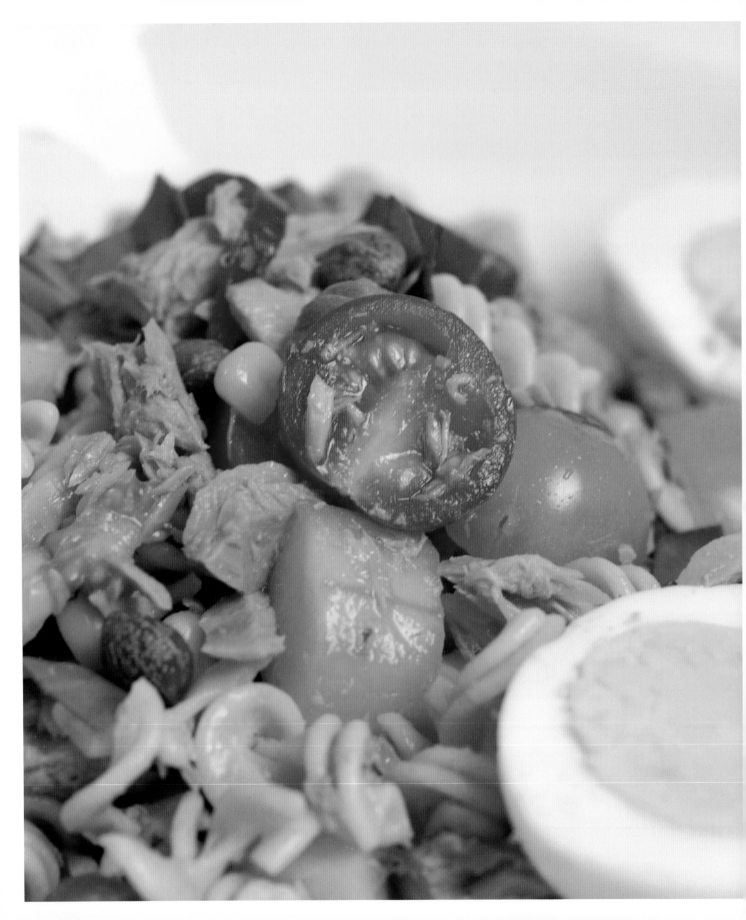

COLORFUL TUNA FUSILLI SALAD

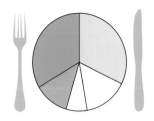

- ▣ Fruit & Vegetables
- ☐ Carbohydrates
- ☐ Milk, Dairy or Alternatives
- ☐ High in Sugar and/or Fat
- ▣ Proteins

This is a flavorful pasta, tuna and vegetables combination – perfect for picnics and barbeques or as a well-balanced main dish. It's packed with proteins, omega-3 essential fats and brilliant flavors making it one of the children's favorite salads too. Nowadays there is a variety of gluten free pastas available in the supermarkets to choose from. For this recipe I like to use brown rice pasta. It's wholegrain and very tasty, not dry and gummy like many other gluten free pastas and above all, absorbs the sauce well. Happy salad assembly!

200 g (7 oz) GF fusilli pasta
150 g (5 oz) canned tuna chunks in olive oil
150 g (5 oz) canned sweet corn
1 handful of fresh basil, finely chopped
1 garlic clove, crushed
1 avocado, sliced
5 cm (2 inches) cucumber, sliced
1 tbsp capers
2 boiled eggs, cut in halves
3 tbsp olive oil
1 tbsp balsamic vinegar
A pinch of salt and freshly ground black pepper to taste

Serves: 2
Preparation Time: 10 min
Cooking Time: 10 min

1. Bring a large pot of lightly salted water to a rapid boil. Add GF fusilli pasta and boil according to the instructions on the packet until al dente (pasta should be cooked to be firm to the bite). To keep pasta from sticking, stir during the first couple of minutes of cooking. Pasta should be ready in around 10 minutes. Once ready, drain the pasta using a fine-mesh strainer and put aside to cool.
2. In a large bowl, add all the ingredients (tuna chunks, sweet corn, basil, garlic, avocado, cucumber, capers, eggs) and toss together.
3. Add fusilli, olive oil and balsamic vinegar and toss it again. Season with salt and pepper and serve immediately.

CORN AND COD SOUP

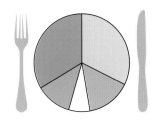

■ Fruit & Vegetables
□ Carbohydrates
■ Milk, Dairy or Alternatives
□ High in Sugar and/or Fat
■ Proteins

This light and easy to make Asian-inspired soup is bursting with masses of nutrients and flavors. The sweetness of sweet corn combined with the subtle flavor of the cod and aromatic flavors of herbs make this dish one of my favorite soups of all time.

Cod is an excellent source of easily digestible proteins, iodine, selenium and B vitamins while sweet corn is packed with magnesium, manganese and C vitamins. This is a soup for all seasons and is best served as a wonderfully delicious appetizer or as an indulgent and flavorful main course. It only takes 15 minutes to make – so no excuses really. Let's get cooking!

....

1 tbsp olive oil
1 red onion, finely chopped
2 garlic cloves, finely chopped
1 lemon grass stalk (whole)
1 cm (½ in) piece fresh ginger, finely chopped
200 ml (7 fl oz) coconut milk (light)
500 ml (17 fl oz) vegetable stock
1 tbsp corn flour
110 g (4 oz) frozen kernels
250 g (9 oz) cod fillet (cut in chunks)
1 tbsp fish sauce
½ lime (juice)
1 handful fresh cilantro (coriander), finely chopped

Serves: 2
Preparation Time: 10 min
Cooking Time: 15 min

1. Heat the olive oil in a casserole type saucepan on a medium heat and gently fry the red onion, garlic, lemon grass and ginger for 2 minutes or until soft and golden brown.
2. Add the coconut milk and vegetable stock and bring to a boil.
3. In separate small bowl, mix the corn flour with two tablespoons of water.
4. Add the frozen corn kernels and corn flour mixture to the casserole saucepan, reduce the heat and simmer gently for 3 minutes.
5. Add the cod cut in chunks, fish sauce and lime juice and simmer gently for 10 minutes. Discard the lemon grass stalk.
6. Ladle into bowls and garnish with finely chopped cilantro.
7. Serve warm.

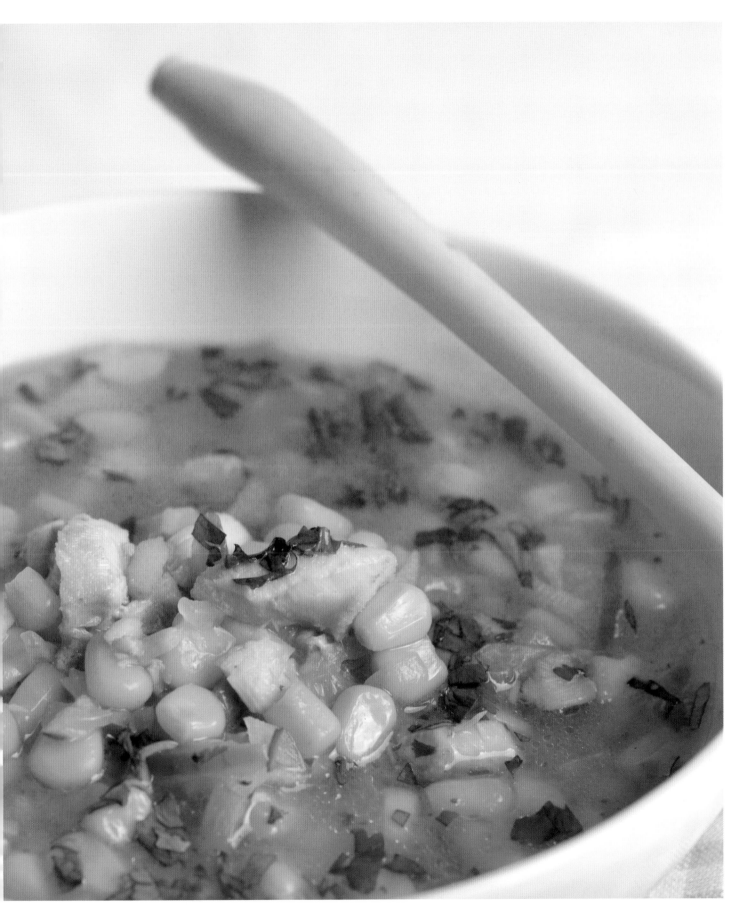

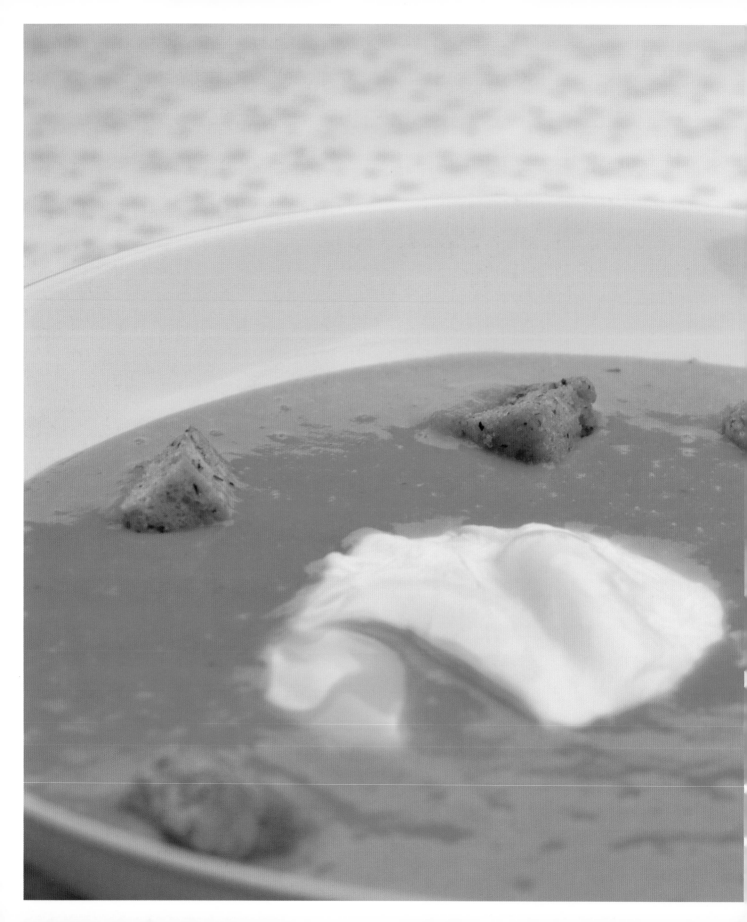

CREAMY ASPARAGUS
AND KALE SOUP

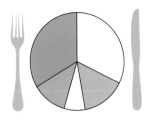

□ Fruit & Vegetables
□ Carbohydrates
□ Milk, Dairy or Alternatives
□ High in Sugar and/or Fat
□ Proteins

This nutritious and comforting asparagus and kale soup is a delight with crunchy gluten free croutons and a protein rich poached egg. The combination of the ingredients in this dish works beautifully together making this dish one of my favorite starters on those cold winter days. My children and some of my dear guests do get put off a bit by its green color to start with but once they taste it, they all get nicely surprised. So come on – go ahead and make this fabulous healthy soup that all family will devour. It's green but it's very tasty!

150 g (5 oz) kale, chopped
3 potatoes, sliced
2 tbsp olive oil
1 white onion, finely sliced
2 sprigs fresh tarragon
1 garlic clove, finely chopped
250 g (9 oz) asparagus
200 ml (7 fl oz) vegetable stock
100 ml (3.5 fl oz) light coconut milk
4 eggs (one per bowl)
a pinch of salt and pepper
GF croutons (optional)

Serves: 4
Preparation Time: 10 min
Cooking Time: 20 min

1. In a medium size saucepan, boil the kale and potatoes for 10 minutes and put aside.
2. Heat the olive oil in a medium pot over medium heat, add sliced onions and gently fry until the onion has softened (fry for about 5 minutes).
3. Add the chopped tarragon and garlic, stir gently for a couple of minutes and then add potatoes, kale, asparagus, vegetable stock and coconut milk.
4. Bring to a boil, reduce the heat, cover and simmer for about 10–15 minutes or until all the vegetables are soft.
5. Pour the mixture into a blender and blend the soup until silky smooth, strain and add a poached egg to each bowl and serve warm.
6. Best served with a handful of crunchy GF croutons. Highly nutritious and delicious!

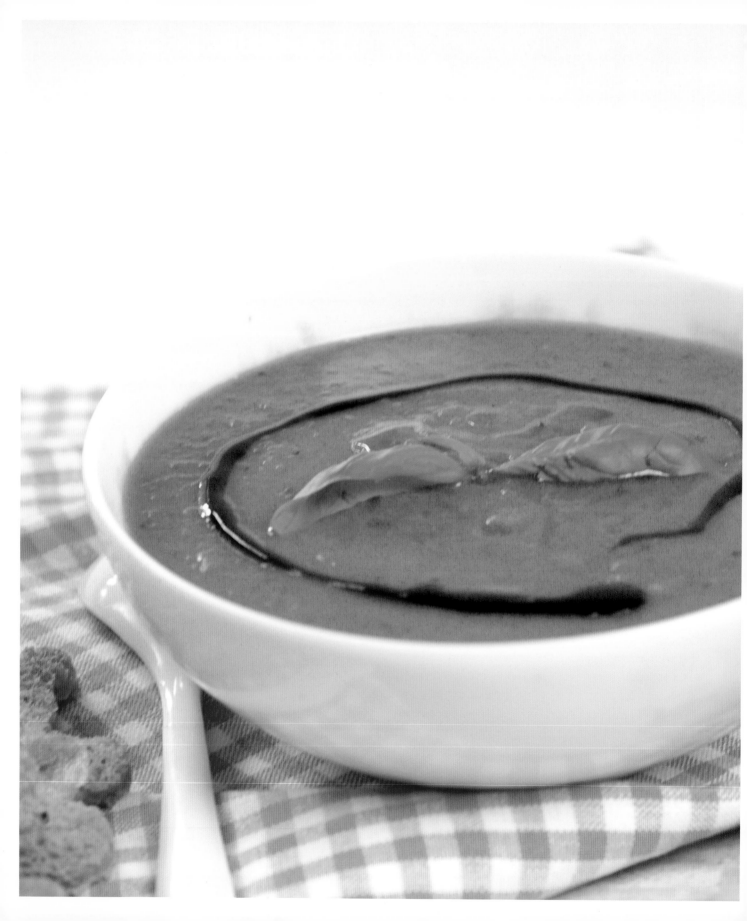

ROASTED CARROTS, LENTILS AND BUTTERNUT SQUASH SOUP

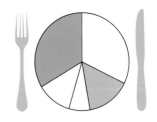

☑ Fruit & Vegetables
☐ Carbohydrates
☑ Milk, Dairy or Alternatives
☐ High in Sugar and/or Fat
☐ Proteins

This is a wonderfully flavorsome soup, rich in proteins and protective antioxidants. The roasting of garlic, carrots, butternut squash and cherry tomatoes brings out the smoky sweetness of this dish that my guests adore.

1 large butternut squash, diced
2 carrots, diced
5 cherry tomatoes
3 garlic cloves
1 tbsp olive oil
1 red onion, finely chopped
300 g (10.5 oz) red lentils
1 tsp sweet paprika
1 liter (1 ¾ pint) vegetable stock
　(made with stock cubes or
　bouillon powder)
50 ml (1.5 fl oz) coconut cream
pinch of salt and pepper

Serves: 6
Preparation Time: 15 min
Cooking Time: 30 min

1.　Preheat the oven to 190°C (375°F).
2.　Place the diced butternut squash, carrots, cherry tomatoes and garlic cloves in a baking tray, drizzle with olive oil, sprinkle with salt and pepper and roast in the oven for 25 minutes or until golden brown.
3.　Heat 1 tablespoon of the olive oil in a large pot, add finely chopped onions and cook until softened. Add the roasted squash, garlic, cherry tomatoes and carrots and then add the lentils and paprika. Mix thoroughly. Pour in vegetable stock, cover and simmer until the lentils are cooked, stirring occasionally.
4.　Season with salt and pepper. Transfer the mixture to a blender and process to a soup of preferred consistency (add more stock if the soup is too thick).
5.　Transfer the blended mixture back in the pan, add the coconut cream and simmer for a further 5 minutes.
6.　Serve warm.

MAMMA'S MINESTRONE

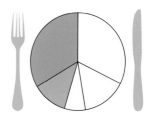

I've got my dear Italian mother-in-law to thank for this delicious soup which is bursting with protective antioxidants and healthy fiber. This is a 'must have' dish in her house and everyone I know loves it. The recipe's been improvised a bit, but the fundamentals are still the same. It does take time to prepare it but all the effort is definitely worth it in the end and, always, try to prepare a bigger batch so you can keep it refrigerated for up to two days or you can freeze it for later use. This is also one of the best ways I know to encourage your children to eat more vegetables. You can also add some gluten free pasta to it to make it a bit richer and thicker. Utterly delicious!

■ Fruit & Vegetables
☐ Carbohydrates
☐ Milk, Dairy or Alternatives
☐ High in Sugar and/or Fat
■ Proteins

3 tbsp olive oil
1 red onion
3 garlic cloves, finely chopped
1 handful of fresh parsley, finely
    chopped
1 handful of fresh basil, finely
    chopped
3 tbsp tomato puree
3 white potatoes
300 g (10.5 oz) fresh carrots
150 g (5 oz) fresh celery
200 g (7 oz) trimmed fresh green
    beans
2.25 liter (4 pint) vegetable stock
400 g (14 oz) borlotti beans
    (canned)
pinch of salt

Serves: 6
Preparation Time: 30 min
Cooking Time: 90 min

1. Place red onion, garlic, parsley and basil in a food processor and finely chop.
2. In a large cooking pot, heat the olive oil on a medium heat, add the chopped vegetables mixture and cook for 5 minutes, stirring occasionally.
3. Add tomato puree to the mixture and cook for a further 5 minutes, stirring occasionally.
4. Add the cut potatoes, carrots, celery and green beans to the pot and pour the vegetable stock over the mixture. Cover the pot, bring to the boil and cook for 20 minutes on a medium heat.
5. Add the canned borlotti beans, reduce heat to low, cover the pot and cook for a further 40 minutes stirring occasionally.
6. Remove the lid and cook for another 10–20 minutes or until you get preferred consistency.
7. If you prefer your soup to be very thick and hearty, leave it cooking on a low heat for a further 15 minutes.
8. Serve warm with or without GF spaghetti or any GF pasta of your choice.

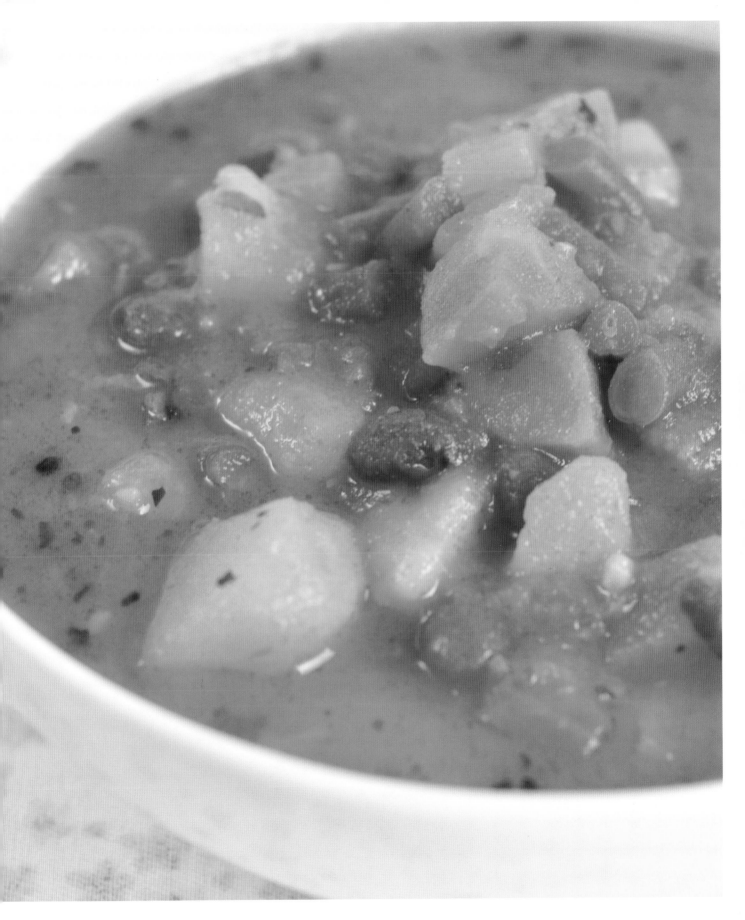

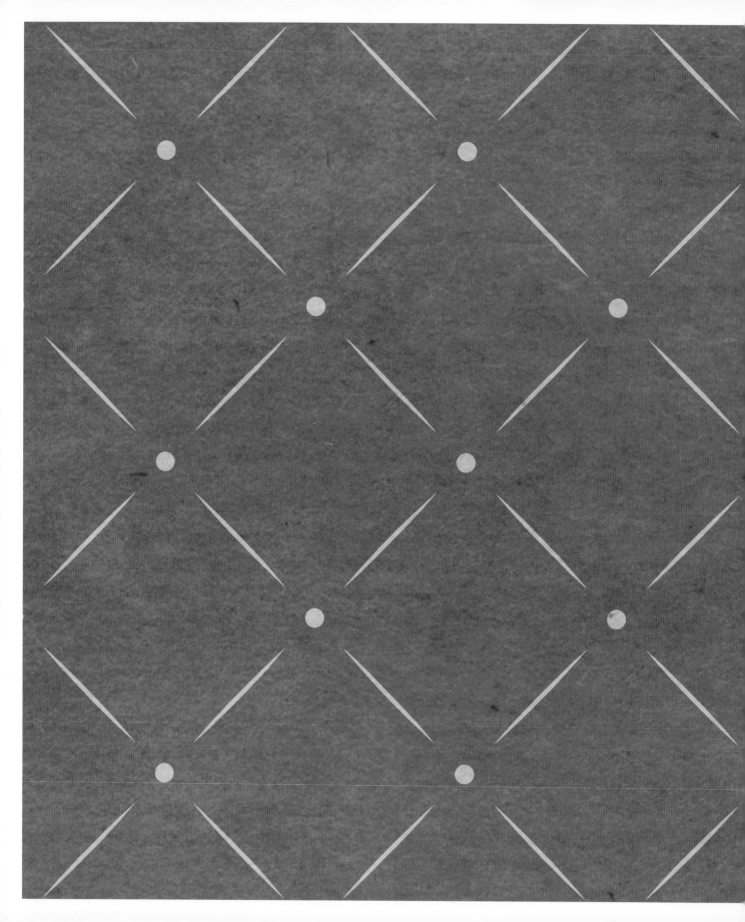

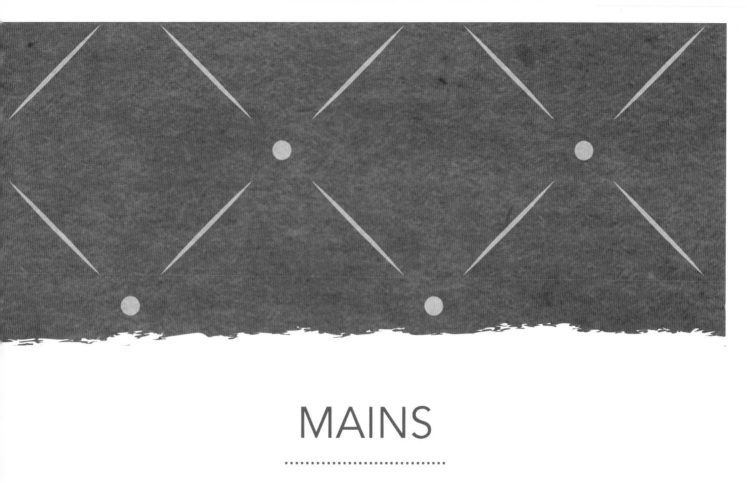

MAINS

·····························

Meat

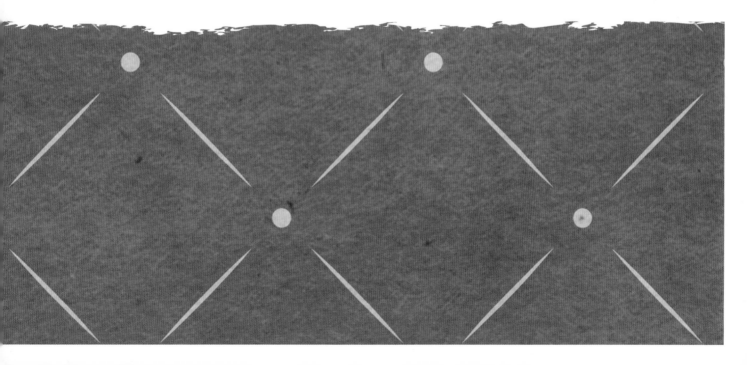

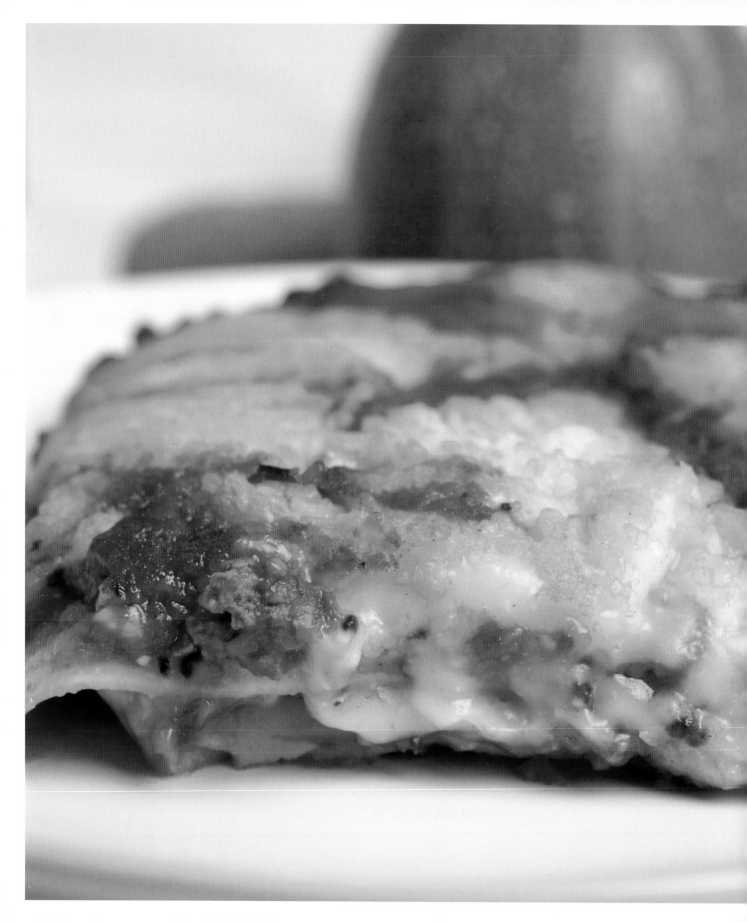

BEEF LASAGNE

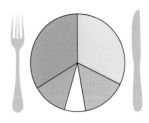

This is a healthy alternative to the calorie-laden traditional cheesy lasagne. Packed with a nutritious lean beef (preferably organic) and topped with a delicious and creamy coconut béchamel, the tastiness of this dish will nicely surprise all traditional lasagne lovers. You will not even realize that all those rich layers of cheese are not even there. It really is a delicious, flavorful and healthy energy booster, and an important source of iron, protein, zinc and B vitamins. So now, if you have your friends over for lunch and you know that they love lasagne, there really is no reason not to make it just because you cannot eat dairies and gluten. Experiment and enjoy!

- ▣ Fruit & Vegetables
- ☐ Carbohydrates
- ▣ Milk, Dairy or Alternatives
- ☐ High in Sugar and/or Fat
- ▣ Proteins

2 tbsp olive oil
400 g (14 oz) lean minced beef
  (10% fat)
2 garlic cloves
1 carrot
1 zucchini (courgette)
1 red onion
1 tbsp chopped parsley
1 tbsp chopped basil
600 ml (1 pint) fresh tomato sauce
  (see page 45)
500 g (1 lb 2 oz) GF lasagne sheets*
500 ml (17 fl oz) béchamel (see
  page 47)
salt and black pepper

Serves: 6
Preparation Time: 30 min
Cooking Time: 35 min

1. Preheat the oven at 190°C (375°F).
2. Add the olive oil to a large casserole-type pan, heat on medium heat and add the minced beef, season with salt and pepper and gently fry for about 10 minutes or until meat starts separating.
3. Finely chop garlic, carrot, zucchini, red onion, parsley and basil and mix well in a separate bowl.
4. Add the vegetable mixture to the meat, mix and gently fry for 5 minutes. Add the tomato sauce and stir for a couple of minutes.
5. To assemble the lasagne, rub an earthenware lasagne dish with olive oil, lay the dish with the lasagne sheets over the bottom and drape the sheets over the sides. Add a layer of meat, vegetables and tomato sauce mixture, then a layer of béchamel and cover it with the lasagne sheet. Repeat the layers until you fill the dish. Always cover with the lasagne sheet on the top.
6. Cook in the preheated oven for 30–35 minutes until golden.
7. Serve warm.

*Please note some brands require pre-cooking, please check instructions on the pack.

CHICKEN CACCIATORE

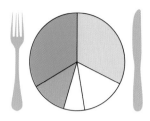

This beautiful chicken cacciatore is a healthy and delicious alternative to traditional Sunday roasts. It's a simple combination of flavors that just work really well and smells heavenly too. Whenever possible, choose organic or free range chicken as these are generally leaner and contain a greater proportion of omega–3 and 6 fats. It's a versatile dish, perfect for social gatherings and can be served on its own or with rice or gluten free pasta. It does require a little work but it's definitely worth it. It can also be kept in the fridge for up to three days. This dish is very popular with my children so I tend to conveniently serve it a couple of days in a row with either pasta or rice.

■ Fruit & Vegetables
□ Carbohydrates
□ Milk, Dairy or Alternatives
□ High in Sugar and/or Fat
■ Proteins

1 tbsp olive oil
6 corn-fed chicken thighs
1 red onion
3 garlic cloves
handful of fresh basil, finely chopped
handful of fresh scented thyme
3 tbsp tomato puree
1.5 liter (2½ pint) water
2 large carrots, thickly sliced
2 zucchinis (courgettes), thickly sliced
2 white potatoes, cubed
1 sweet potato
salt and pepper

Serves: 6
Preparation Time: 20 min
Cooking Time: 60 min

1. In a casserole pan, heat the olive oil on a medium heat, add the chicken thighs and gently fry until golden brown on both sides.
2. Add the chopped onion, garlic, basil and fresh thyme, mix thoroughly and cook for further 5 minutes.
3. Stir in the tomato puree, mix again and continue cooking for another 3 minutes.
4. In a separate pan, bring about 1.5 liters of water to a boil.
5. Cut all the vegetables into chunks and add them to the casserole mix. Pour boiling water into the casserole pan, season well with the salt and pepper.
6. Reduce the heat and simmer for around 60 minutes.
7. Serve warm.

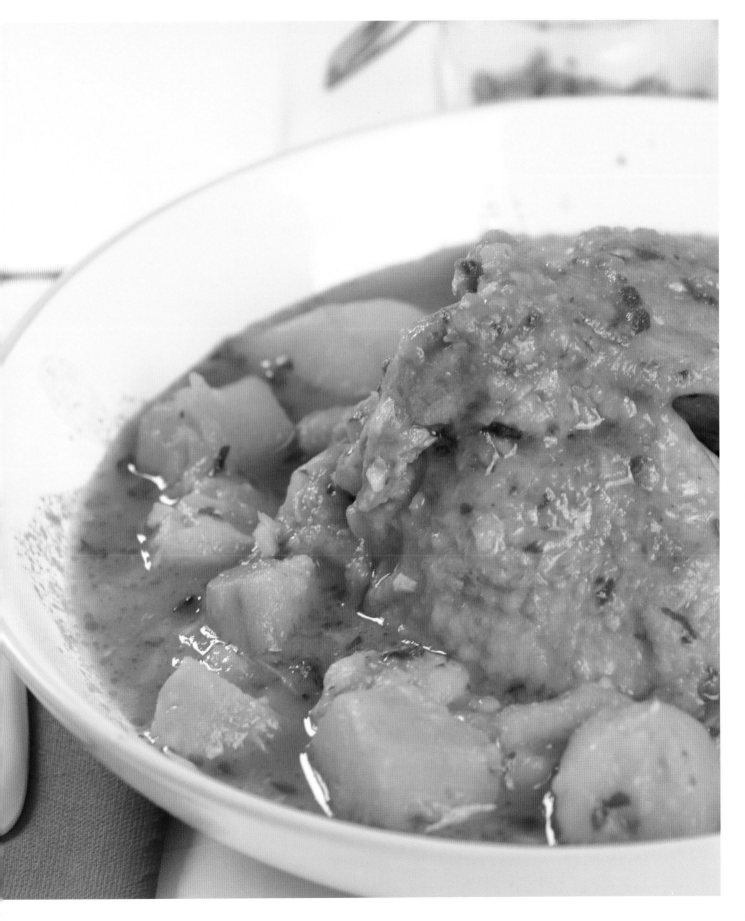

LIGHT CHICKEN STEW WITH CORN FLOUR DUMPLINGS

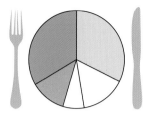

This light and comforting stew is rich in flavor and essential nutrients. A perfect dish for those long and cold wintery days when your body is calling for a meal that is warm and filling. Chicken is low in saturated fats and rich in proteins and minerals, especially the mineral selenium, which is essential for a healthy immune system. As with all other meats, whenever possible, buy organic or free range chickens as these are generally leaner and tastier. On the other hand, corn is a good source of dietary fiber, iron and phosphorus and is also naturally gluten free. This aromatic, no fuss stew is a perfect healthy alternative to either fish and chips on Fridays or roast lunch on Sundays. Let's be a bit more adventurous.

■ Fruit & Vegetables
□ Carbohydrates
□ Milk, Dairy or Alternatives
□ High in Sugar and/or Fat
■ Proteins

Chicken Stew:

1 tbsp olive oil
1 onion, finely chopped
2 garlic cloves, finely chopped
2 carrots, cubed
4 chicken drumsticks or thighs
2 branches of fresh thyme
1 tbsp fresh parsley
1.2 liter (2 pint) vegetable stock
salt and freshly ground black pepper

Dumplings:

8 tbsp corn flour
1 egg
2 tbsp water
2 tbsp olive oil
Salt to taste

Serves: 4
Preparation Time: 15 min
Cooking Time: 40 min

1. In a large casserole type pan, heat the olive oil on a medium heat. Add onion, garlic and carrots and gently fry for 3 minutes, stirring occasionally.
2. Add chicken thighs and/or drumsticks (you may want to use wings or chicken breast instead) and cook until chicken is golden brown on all sides. Add thyme and parsley and mix thoroughly. Pour in the hot vegetable stock, season with salt and freshly ground black pepper, increase heat to high and bring to the boil. Boil for 30 minutes or until the chicken is cooked through.
3. Meanwhile, prepare the dumplings: in a small bowl combine, corn flour, the egg, water and olive oil and mix well with a fork until well blended. The batter should not be too thick– it should easily drop from the tip of the spoon. If too thick, add some more water.
4. Drop the dumpling batter a teaspoon at a time into the simmering chicken broth, cover and cook for 7–10 minutes or until the dumplings are cooked through. Ensure that the dumplings are well spaced apart as they expand during the cooking process.
5. Once the dumplings are ready, remove from the heat, garnish with fresh parsley and serve immediately.

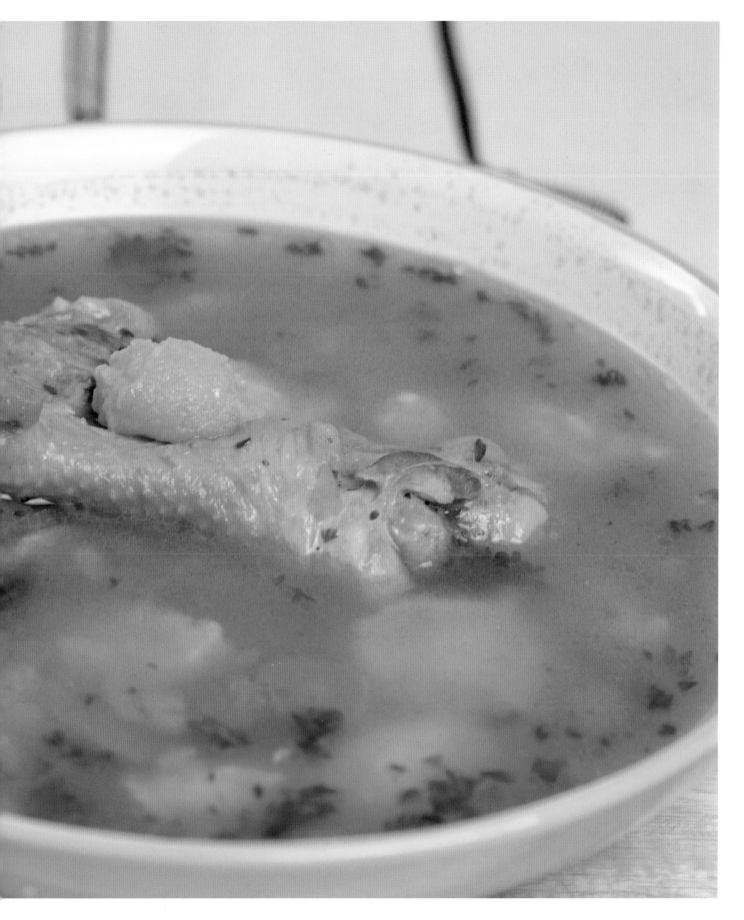

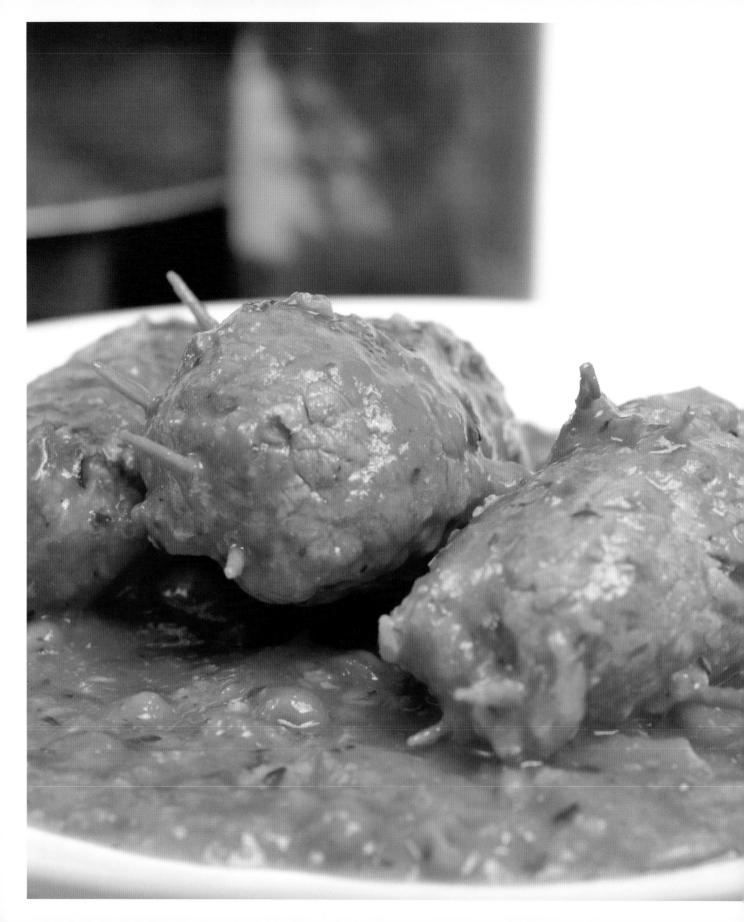

STUFFED VEAL ROLLS

This vibrant and sophisticated dish is full of the Mediterranean flavors that will, in no time, bring you back to charming Southern Italy. Rich and sweet tomato sauce, tangy green olives, and the strong savory flavor of anchovies blend perfectly with lean, organic and flavorful veal making this dish one of my family's favorites. The addition of anchovies makes the meat even meatier. For a vegetarian version of the dish, you can easily substitute veal escalope with thin, lengthwise, slices of grilled eggplants. This really is a dish to impress. While it looks interesting on a plate, it's also packed with masses of nutrients and flavor. Veal is an excellent source of iron, proteins, B vitamins and zinc. Anchovies are rich in omega-3 fatty acids and vitamin A, while tomato sauce is a good source of antioxidant lycopene and vitamin C. It does take a bit longer to prepare but all the effort is well worth it in the end. It's best served with a crunchy salad but if you are really hungry, you can have it with rice or quinoa.

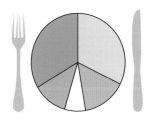

- ■ Fruit & Vegetables
- □ Carbohydrates
- □ Milk, Dairy or Alternatives
- □ High in Sugar and/or Fat
- ■ Proteins

Serves: 4
Preparation Time: 20 min
Cooking Time: 45 min

* * *

650g (1 lb 5 oz) veal escalope
    (8 x 80 g slices)
80 g (3 oz) cooked ham
30 g (1 oz) green olives, finely
    chopped
1 garlic clove, finely chopped
1 tbsp parsley, finely chopped
1 egg
1 tbsp anchovy paste
30 g (1 oz) brown rice flour
2 tbsp olive oil
1 carrot, julienned
400 ml (14 fl oz) vegetable stock
1 tsp corn flour
20 g (0.75 oz) sweet peas
    (frozen or fresh)
2 tbsp coconut cream
2 tbsp tomato sauce
freshly ground black pepper to
    taste

1. Place each veal slice (1 x 70 g/2.5 oz) between two sheets of plastic wrap and bash with a meat mallet or a rolling pin until very thin.
2. In a large ball, combine the finely chopped ham, green olives, garlic and parsley. Add one egg, anchovy paste, tomato sauce and rice flour. Mix well and season with black pepper. Do not add salt at this point as the anchovy paste and green olives are already quite salty.
3. Place a tablespoonful of the mixture in the center of each thinned beef slice (escalope) and roll up tightly, sealing in the mixture.
4. Secure the rolls firmly with cocktail sticks or kitchen strings.
5. Add the olive oil to a casserole type saucepan and heat on a medium heat. Add the meat rolls and gently fry for 2–3 minutes until browned on all sides.
6. Add the julienned carrots and the vegetable stock and simmer for 40 minutes or until the stock has evaporated by half.
7. In a separate small bowl, mix 1 teaspoon of corn flour with 2 tablespoons of water and add the mixture into the saucepan. Stir in the sweet peas and coconut cream and reduce further until the sauce thickens.
8. Serve warm with crunchy salad, rice or quinoa.

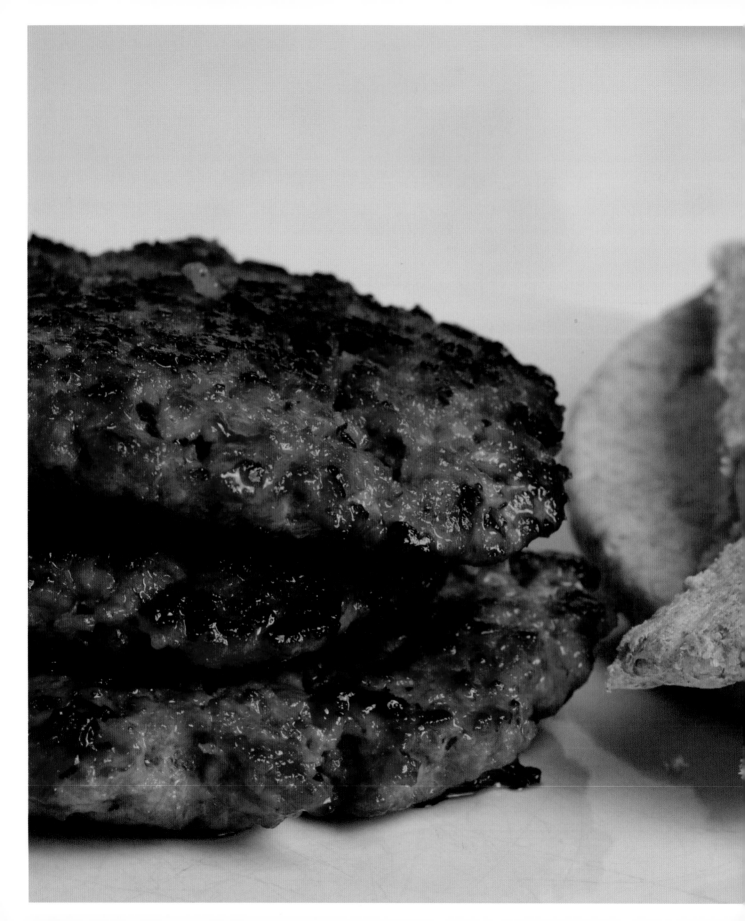

SUCCULENT PORK AND VEAL BURGERS

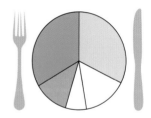

One thing I like about homemade burgers is that you know exactly what is in them – you know that if you buy fresh organic or free range meat your burgers will be richer in nutrients, less fattening and above all, will definitely taste better. You also know that you can always tweak the recipe until you get your best burger ever. This is exactly what has happened here: the combination of the ingredients in this recipe works perfectly. Slightly sweet pork blends beautifully with lean beef to make these wonderfully moist burgers that all the family will enjoy. Not only do they taste heavenly, they are also good for you: the mince is packed with proteins, iron, zinc and B12 vitamins that facilitates production of the red blood cells in the body and is an excellent source of energy while garlic is well known for its antimicrobial properties. Who said burgers were bad for you especially when served with beautiful fresh and crispy salad?

- ■ Fruit & Vegetables
- ☐ Carbohydrates
- ☐ Milk, Dairy or Alternatives
- ☐ High in Sugar and/or Fat
- ■ Proteins

....

300 g (10.5 oz) minced veal
200 g (7 oz) minced pork
30 g (2 oz) GF breadcrumbs
1 tsp tomato paste
1 tbsp basil, finely chopped
1 tbsp parsley, finely chopped
1 garlic clove, finely chopped
1 shallot, finely chopped
salt and freshly ground black pepper
    to season

Serves: 4
Preparation Time: 10 min +
15 min chilling
Cooking Time: 5 min

1. Preheat the grill to medium.
2. Put the pork and beef mince, GF breadcrumbs, tomato paste and finely chopped basil, shallot, parsley and garlic in a large bowl season with salt and freshly ground black pepper and gently mix together with your hands.
3. Shape the mixture into around 10 burgers (you can make more or less than this, depending on what size burgers you prefer), line them on a plate and put them in the fridge to chill for about 15–30 minutes.
4. Lightly grease a grill grate and grill the burgers for about 4–5 minutes on each side or until golden brown.
5. Serve warm.

SUPER QUICK AND HEALTHY CHICKEN NUGGETS

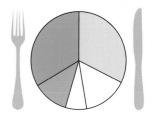

- ■ Fruit & Vegetables
- ☐ Carbohydrates
- ☐ Milk, Dairy or Alternatives
- ☐ High in Sugar and/or Fat
- ■ Proteins

This is a healthy and delicious alternative to fast-food, breaded and deep fried chicken nuggets. In fact, this is as healthy as chicken nuggets can really get – no breading or battering and no deep-frying either. And it gets better – my children absolutely love them! Whenever possible, use an organic chicken breast as it definitely tastes better and is a lot leaner too. To add sweetness to it, simply combine it with organic carrots and simmer it in a flavorful tomato sauce. Chicken is a good source of protein while carrots are rich in antioxidants and soluble fiber.

This super quick and simple dish is irresistibly delicious. Sometimes we really don't need to spend hours in the kitchen to prepare a meal that everyone will talk about.

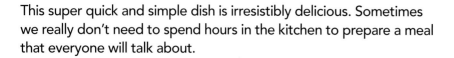

300 g (10.5 oz) organic chicken breast, cubed
½ carrot, cut into chunks
1 tbsp brown rice flour
1 egg
500 ml (17 fl oz) tomato sauce (see page 45 or use any readymade tomato sauce)
100 ml (3.5 fl oz) water
2 tbsp olive oil
1 pinch of salt

Serves: 4
Preparation Time: 5 min
Cooking Time: 15 min

1. Place the chicken cubes and carrot chunks into an electric chopper and process to form a thick paste.
2. Transfer the mixture into a medium size bowl, add one tablespoon of brown rice flour (or you can use any other GF flour), and an egg, season with salt and mix thoroughly.
3. Heat the olive oil in a large saucepan on a medium heat.
4. Shape the mixture into an oval shape. Form the dumpling using two tablespoons – put the dollop of the mixture into one tablespoon and roll the mixture from one spoon to the other to form an oval shape dumpling.
5. Transfer the dumplings into the large saucepan and gently fry for 5 minutes or until lightly browned.
6. Add the tomato sauce and water, mix thoroughly and gently simmer for a further 10 minutes. If the sauce thickens too quickly, add a bit more water.
7. Serve warm with crunchy salad.

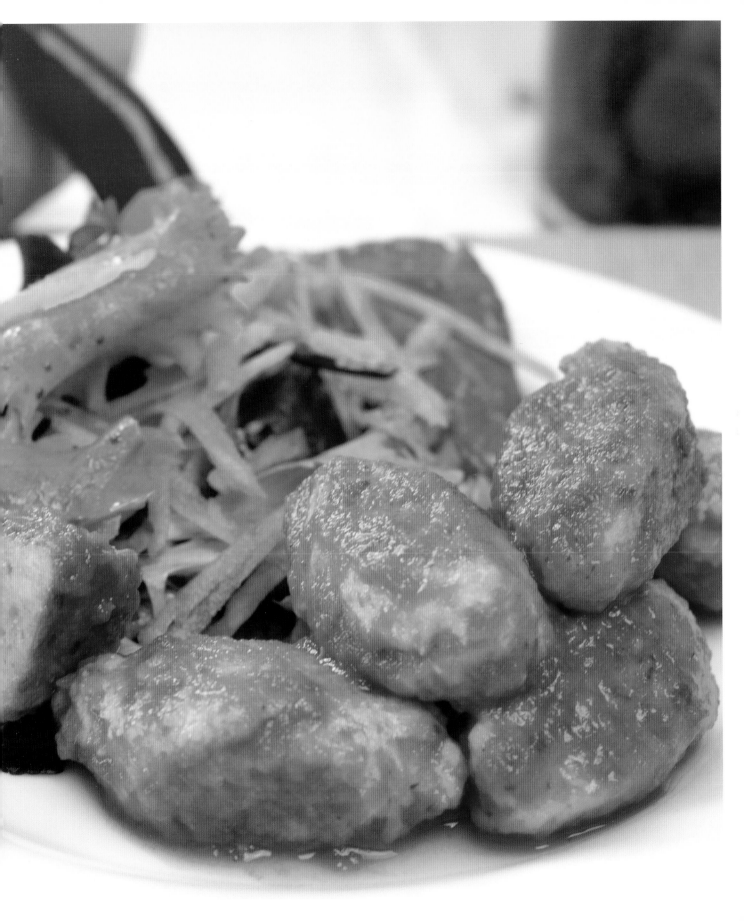

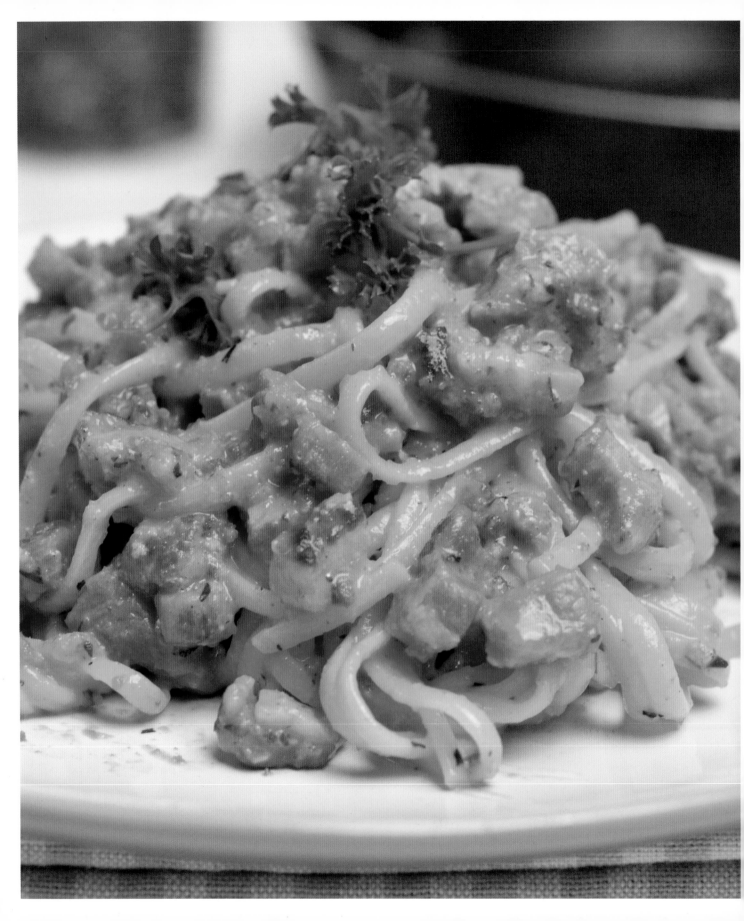

LIGUINI ALLA CARBONARA

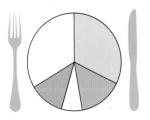

☐ Fruit & Vegetables
☐ Carbohydrates
☑ Milk, Dairy or Alternatives
☐ High in Sugar and/or Fat
☑ Proteins

This book wouldn't be complete without linguini alla carbonara. This irresistibly delicious Italian-inspired dish is a winner every time. The key to make it work well is the quality of the ingredients and a good technique. Always use organic eggs because they taste better and are free of chemicals and genetically modified materials. Ensure that you remember not to cook the egg yolks in a pan, as they will scramble. Only mix the cooked pasta with the egg yolks and bacon mixture and the residual heat will slowly cook the eggs. The pancetta combined with the cream and egg yolks, give it a wonderfully rich and smoky taste.

400 g (14 oz) GF spaghetti
200 g (7 oz) pancetta (Italian bacon), cubed
5 organic egg yolks
2 tbsp coconut cream
60 g (2 oz) pangrattato (see page 46)
Salt and pepper to taste

Serves: 4
Preparation Time: 15 min
Cooking Time: 10 min

1. Place the pancetta cubes onto a non-stick frying pan and gently fry until light brown. Put aside to cool down. In the meantime, fill a deep casserole pan ¾ full with water, add 1 teaspoon of coarse sea salt for every 2 liters of water, and bring to the boil.
2. Add the spaghetti and cook according to the instructions on the packet or until "al dente". Taste the pasta regularly to ensure you do not overcook it.
3. In a large bowl, place the egg yolks, coconut cream, fried pancetta, 40 g (1½ oz) of pangrattato, season with salt and freshly ground black pepper and mix well. Do not cook the mixture as the eggs will scramble.
4. Drain the pasta using a strainer (keep one cup of cooking water aside) and stir quickly into eggs and bacon mixture. Add 2 tablespoons of pasta water to loosen and mix well. The residual heat from the cooked pasta will cook the eggs but work quickly to prevent eggs from scrambling. If dry, add a bit more of the reserved water.
5. Serve immediately and sprinkle with pangrattato for extra taste and flavor.

LAMB NECK AND CAVOLO NERO CASSEROLE

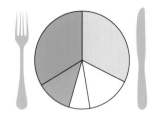

This Italian-inspired, rich and flavorful dish is perfect comfort food on those long and wintery days. It also, very often, reminds me of my mother's cooking when casseroles were 'must have' dishes in the house. Cavolo nero and all other vegetables and seasonings blend perfectly with the rich and strong flavor of succulent lamb fillets. Lamb is an excellent source of iron, protein and energizing B vitamins while cavolo nero (dark-leaved variety of kale from Tuscany) is rich in calcium, fiber and K, A and C vitamins. It does take some time and effort to prepare this hearty dish, but all the effort is definitely worth it in the end. Always try to make a big batch as once ready, you can easily refrigerate if for a couple of days or even freeze it for later use. OK, let's get cooking now – your guests will truly appreciate all your efforts.

■ Fruit & Vegetables
□ Carbohydrates
□ Milk, Dairy or Alternatives
□ High in Sugar and/or Fat
■ Proteins

Serves: 6
Preparation Time: 10 min
Cooking Time: 90 min

---

600 g (1 lb 5 oz) lamb neck fillets, cut into large chunks (organic, if possible)
2 tbsp corn flour
2 tbsp olive oil
1 red onion, finely chopped
3 garlic cloves, finely chopped
1 handful of basil, finely chopped
2 branches of fresh thyme
1 handful of parsley, finely chopped
2 tbsp tomato puree
300 g (10.5 oz) white potatoes, cubed
150 g (5 oz) carrots, cubed
300 g (10.5 oz) cavolo-nero, sliced
1.5 liter (2 ½ pint) vegetable stock
2 bay leaves
1 tsp dry oregano
Salt and freshly ground black pepper to taste

1. Cut the lamb fillets into 2.5 cm (1 inch) chunks.
2. Place the corn flour on a plate and coat each piece of the meat on all sides. The coating will keep the meat moist and adds texture to the sauce.
3. In a high casserole pan, heat the olive oil on a medium heat, add the coated lamb chunks and gently fry until golden brown.
4. Add the chopped onions, garlic, basil, fresh thyme, parsley; mix thoroughly and cook for a further 5 minutes.
5. Stir in the tomato puree, mix again and continue cooking for another 3 minutes.
6. Cube the potatoes and carrots, thickly slice cavolo nero and add into the casserole mixture. Add the vegetable stock, bay leaves, oregano and season with salt and pepper.
7. Cover and cook for 70 minutes on a medium heat, stirring occasionally.
8. Uncover and cook for another 20 minutes to reduce and thicken the sauce.
9. Serve warm with rice.

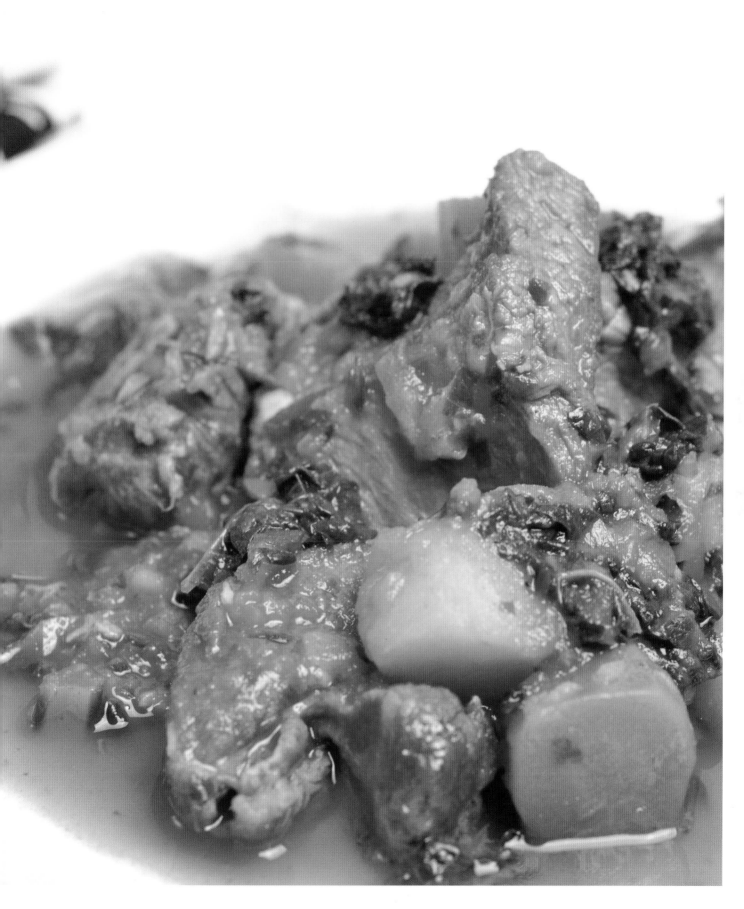

VEAL-STUFFED EGGPLANTS

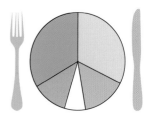

This sophisticated stuffed eggplant dish is a hit with all my guests so far. It looks pretty on a plate, it's packed with masses of nutrients and flavors and it isn't a kind of dish that you will eat every day. It does take some time to prepare, but all the effort is definitely worth it in the end. Eggplants are naturally packed with antioxidants and soluble fiber while veal is rich in proteins, iron and energizing B vitamins. This dish is an excellent energy booster that all the family will enjoy. Now, instead of a usual Sunday roast, why not have these super delicious stuffed eggplants with a crunchy salad on the side instead?
So, please, go ahead and surprise your guests.

■ Fruit & Vegetables
☐ Carbohydrates
■ Milk, Dairy or Alternatives
☐ High in Sugar and/or Fat
■ Proteins

1 large eggplant (aubergine)
1 tbsp olive oil
2 garlic cloves, finely chopped
1 white onion, finely chopped
4 tbsp tomato sauce
30 g (1 oz) coconut cream
1 tbsp fresh basil, finely chopped
1 tsp dry oregano
100 g (3.5 oz) minced veal
1 egg
20 g (0.75 oz) GF breadcrumbs
Salt and freshly ground black pepper

Serves: 2
Preparation Time: 15 min
Cooking Time: 40 min

1. Preheat the oven to 220°C (425°F).
2. Cut eggplant lengthways in half and then carefully cut through the flesh down to the skin, taking care not to cut through the skin.
3. Place them side by side on a baking tray, drizzle with olive oil, season with salt and bake for 30 minutes or until the flesh is soft and tender but not browned.
4. Meanwhile, heat the olive oil in a large non-stick frying pan. Add the chopped garlic and onion and fry gently for 5 minutes, stirring occasionally. Add the tomato sauce, coconut cream, basil, oregano and minced veal, and cook for 10 minutes on a medium heat.
5. Remove the eggplants from the oven and carefully scoop the flesh out of the baked eggplant halves without cutting through the skin.
6. Stir the scooped-out flesh into the veal mixture with a pinch of salt and freshly ground black pepper to taste. Add the beaten egg and mix well.
7. Spoon the mixture into each eggplant shell, sprinkle with GF breadcrumbs, drizzle with a little more olive oil and bake for 15 minutes or until golden brown.
8. Serve warm.

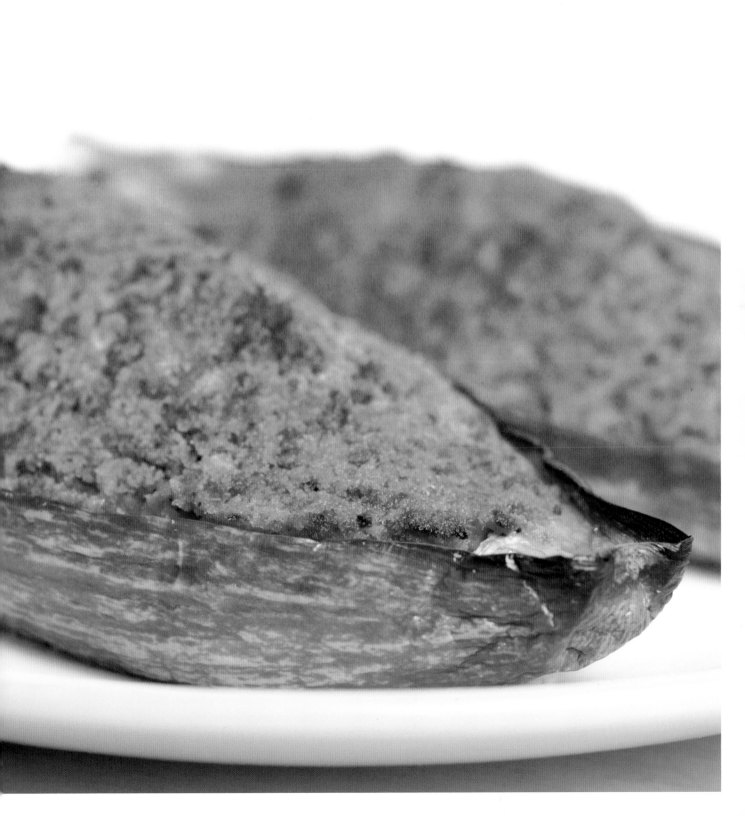

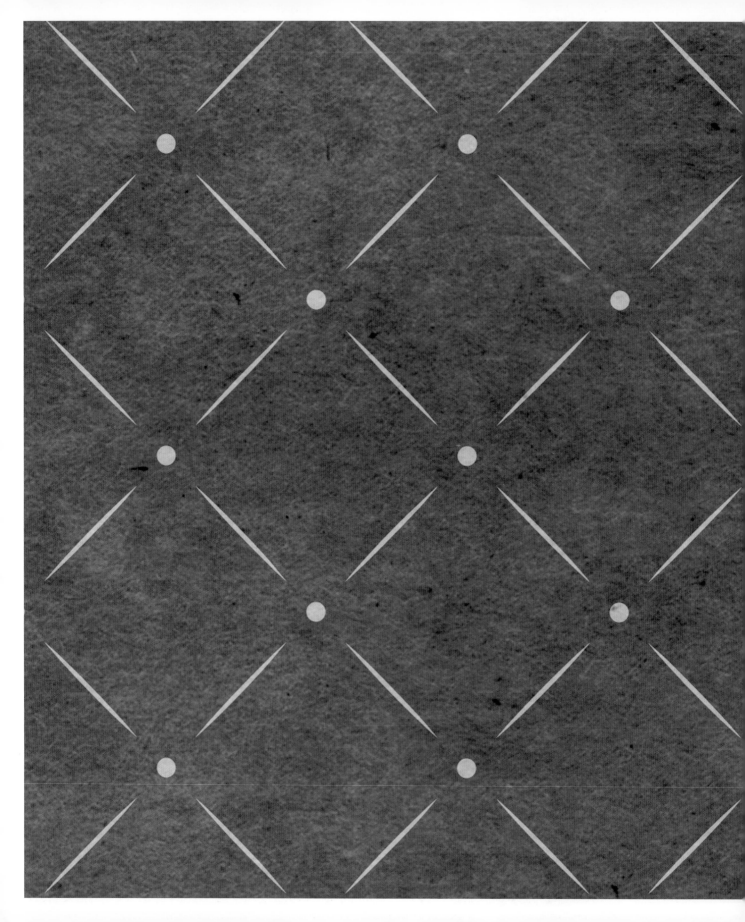

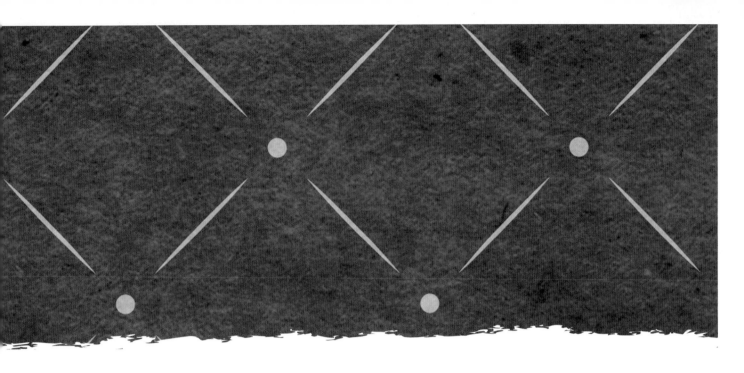

MAINS

·······························

Seafood

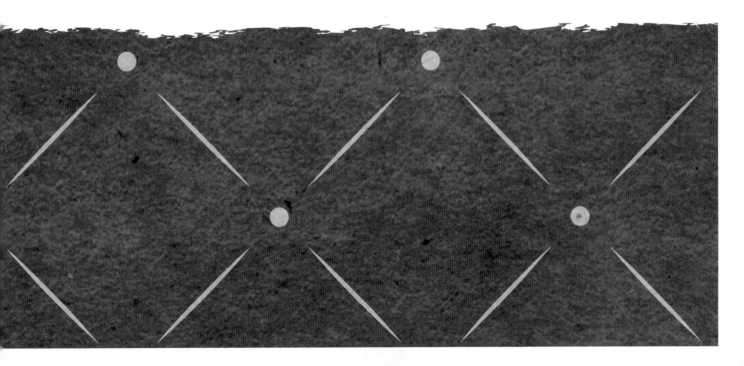

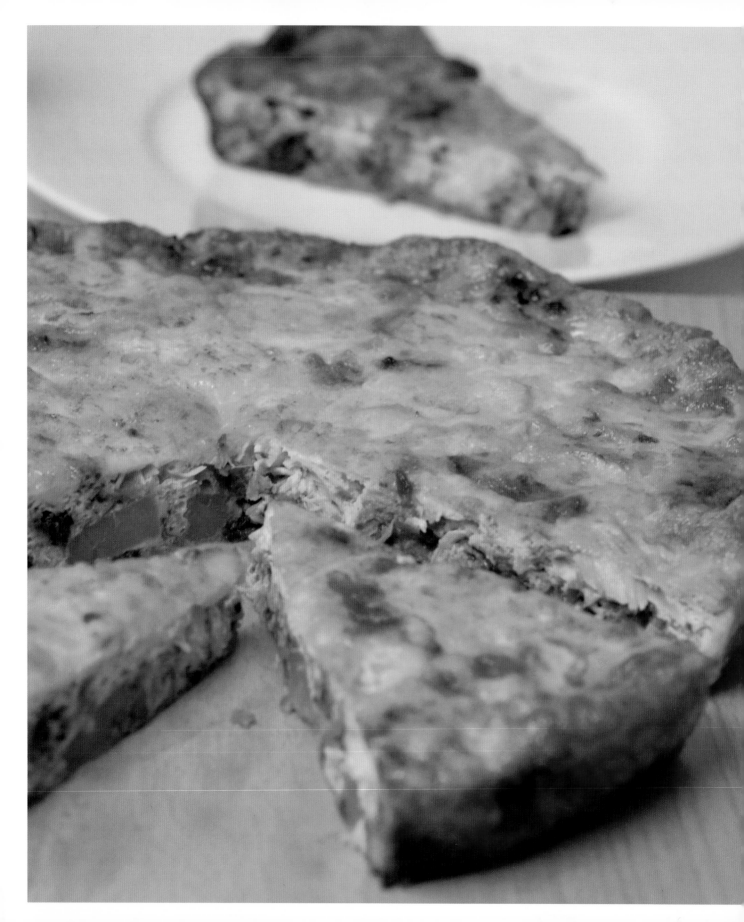

KALE AND SALMON QUICHE

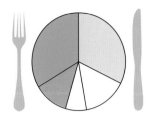

■ Fruit & Vegetables
□ Carbohydrates
□ Milk, Dairy or Alternatives
□ High in Sugar and/or Fat
■ Proteins

This is a delicious, super-healthy dish, bursting with masses of nutrients including omega-3 fatty acids rich salmon, calcium-rich kale, (essential nutrients to include in your diet if you do not eat dairies) and many, many more. And also, this is a quiche with a twist – it does not include pastry as quiches traditionally do, making it an even healthier option for the whole family. It is a perfect choice for school lunch boxes or as a picnic snack. It will keep your little ones fuller for longer but is still light. This is definitely a meal not to be missed!

50 g (1.75 oz) kale
70 g (2.5 oz) asparagus
130 g (4.5 oz) butternut squash
60 ml (2 fl oz) coconut milk
250 g (9 oz) salmon fillet
1 handful of fresh parsley
1 handful of fresh basil
½ red onion
2 tbsp olive oil
1 tbsp coconut oil
4 eggs
170 ml (6 fl oz) coconut cream
100 g (3.5 oz) smoked salmon
1 tbsp tomato paste
Pinch of salt and black pepper

Serves: 6
Preparation Time: 20 min
Cooking Time: 35 min

1. Preheat oven to 200°C (400°F).
2. Cut the vegetables into chunks.
3. Bring a large pot of water to the boil, add kale, asparagus, butternut squash and a bit of salt to enhance the vegetables flavor and boil for 10 minutes.
4. Pour the coconut milk into a medium pot, add a salmon fillet, a few leaves of fresh parsley, season with salt and pepper and bring to boil. As soon as the milk starts boiling, switch off the heat, cover the pot and leave salmon to poach in the milk for 10 minutes.
5. Finely chop parsley, basil and onion, (best done using a mini electric chopper) and fry the mixture in olive oil on low heat for 3 minutes. Add sliced smoked salmon and tomato paste and gently fry for a further 3 minutes.
6. Add the boiled and chunky vegetables into the mixture and fry on a low heat for an additional 10–15 minutes or until the mixture is almost dry (remove as much moisture as possible without over-cooking the vegetables).
7. Grease a tart tray with coconut oil and spread the vegetable mixture evenly.
8. In a medium bowl, whisk the eggs with coconut cream, season with a pinch of salt and pour over the vegetable mixture in the tray.
9. Flake the poached salmon and evenly distribute on top of the mixture
10. Bake in the oven at 200°C (400°F) for 35 minutes. Let it stand for 10 minutes before cutting.

CREAMY POTATO GNOCCHI WITH SALMON AND SWEET PEAS

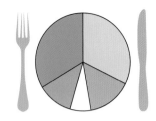

■ Fruit & Vegetables
□ Carbohydrates
■ Milk, Dairy or Alternatives
□ High in Sugar and/or Fat
■ Proteins

Made in minutes, this dish is an absolute winner any time. The smokiness of the salmon blends beautifully with the sweetness of the peas to create this wonderfully creamy and flavorful gnocchi dish. This is a great energy booster rich in proteins, B vitamins and lauric acid from the coconut cream, which is known for its anti-viral and anti-bacterial properties. In fact, this dish is so good it can be a little addictive – just remember not to eat it too fast!

1 tbsp olive oil
2 tbsp chopped shallots
250 g (9 oz) salmon fillets, cubed (2 fillets, preferably lightly smoked if available)
2 tsp chopped fresh basil
1 tsp chopped fresh thyme
3 tbsp tomato sauce
150 ml (5 fl oz) coconut cream
1 sliced sweet chili
150 g (5 oz) frozen sweet peas
500 g (1 lb 2 oz) GF potato gnocchi
Pinch of salt and freshly ground black pepper

Serves: 4
Preparation Time: 10 min
Cooking Time: 10 min

1. Bring a saucepan full of water to boil, add salt.
2. Gently heat the olive oil in a saucepan.
3. Add the shallots and gently fry until soft and golden brown.
4. Add the salmon, chopped basil and thyme. Pour over the tomato sauce and mix well.
5. Cook for a further 3 minutes and then add the coconut cream.
6. In the meantime, pour the peas into the boiling water and leave them for 3 minutes.
7. After 3 minutes, remove the peas from the water with a fine mesh strainer and add them into the saucepan mixture. Make sure to keep the hot water.
8. Add the gnocchi into the same boiling water where you cooked the peas and leave them to boil for a couple of minutes or until they rise to the surface.
9. Once on the surface, remove the gnocchi from the water and gently add them into the saucepan mixture.
10. Mix well and cook for a further couple of minutes on a low heat.
11. Remove from the heat and serve warm.

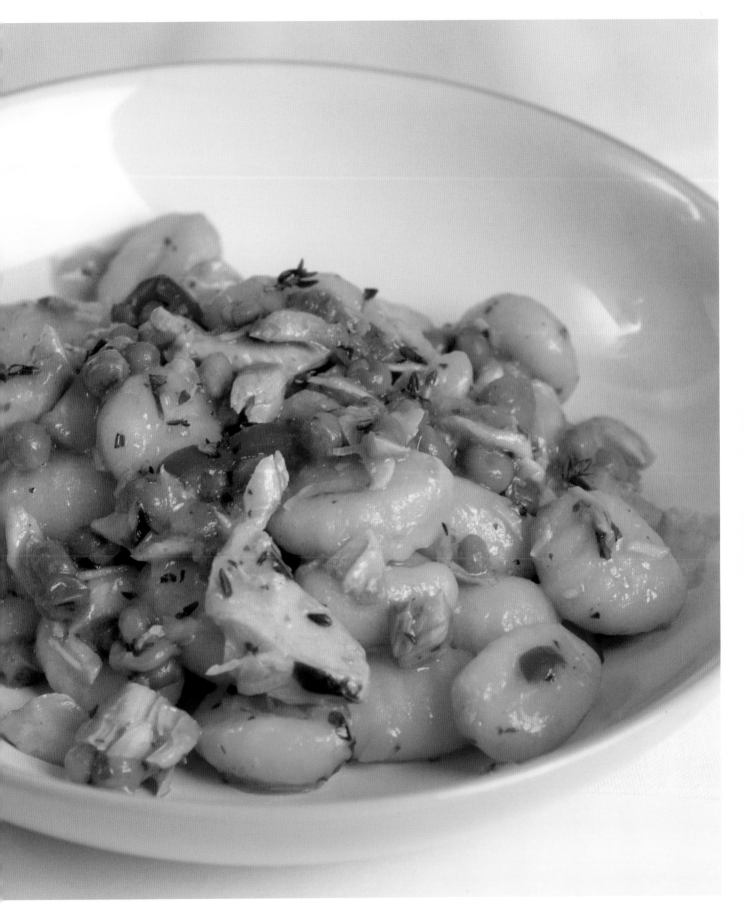

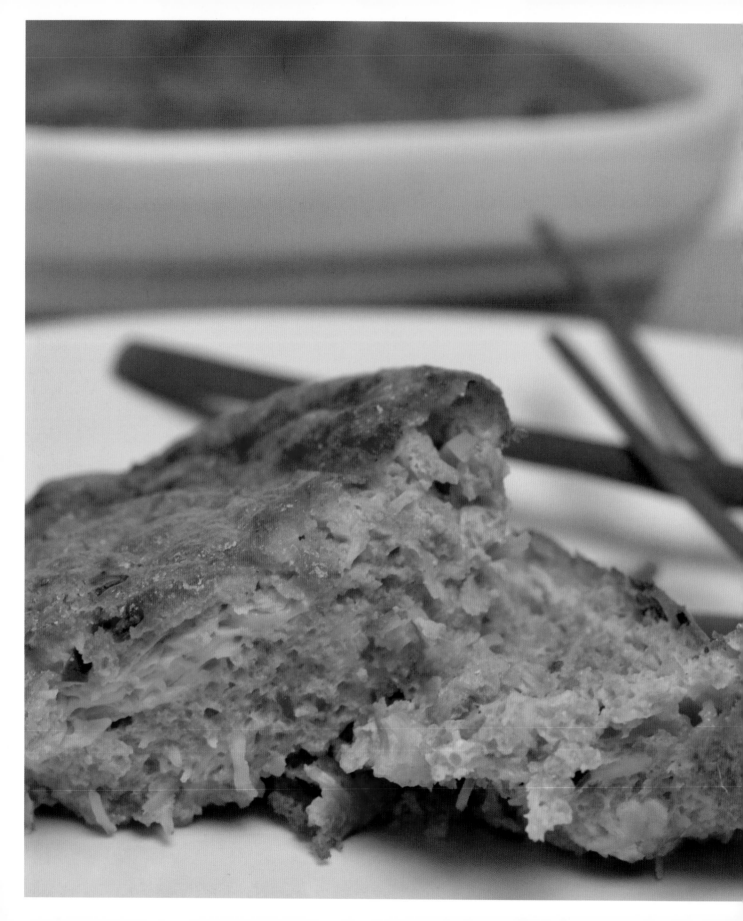

CRAB SOUFFLÉ

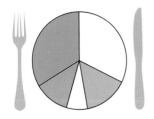

This easy-to-make dish is packed with nutrients and flavor. I very often like to call it 'an omega-3 in a pot' as the crab meat is, indeed, very rich in omega-3 fatty acids. In fact, white and brown crab meat complement each other perfectly. Brown meat has a strong and rich flavor and is packed with omega-3 fatty acids while white meat is rich in proteins, very low in fat and has a milder and more distinctive flavor. Eggs, on the other hand, are a complete source of protein and are rich in vitamin D, iron, vitamin B12 and other nutrients. This flavorsome dish is best served warm with a vibrant salad on the side. I prefer to use small ramekins when baking this dish so that each of my family or friends gets one individual ramekin shaped portion that looks very presentable on a plate.

□ Fruit & Vegetables
□ Carbohydrates
□ Milk, Dairy or Alternatives
□ High in Sugar and/or Fat
□ Proteins

4 eggs
2 tbsp chives, finely chopped
40 ml (1.5 fl oz) light coconut milk
1 tsp corn flour
100 g (3.5 oz) crab meat, white and brown, cooked and shredded
80 ml (3 fl oz) coconut cream
1 tsp olive oil
Salt and freshly ground black pepper

Serves: 4
Preparation Time: 10 min
Cooking Time: 45 min

1. In a medium size bowl, add eggs, light coconut milk (reserving 2 tablespoons), and chopped chives and mix well.
2. In a separate small bowl, add one teaspoon of corn flour and mix with 2 tablespoons of coconut milk and, add to the mixture.
3. Stir in the crab meat and coconut cream, season with salt and pepper and mix gently.
4. Pour the mixture into four greased baking ramekins or two small baking pots.
5. Bake for 40 minutes and serve warm on its own or with a vibrant salad on the side.

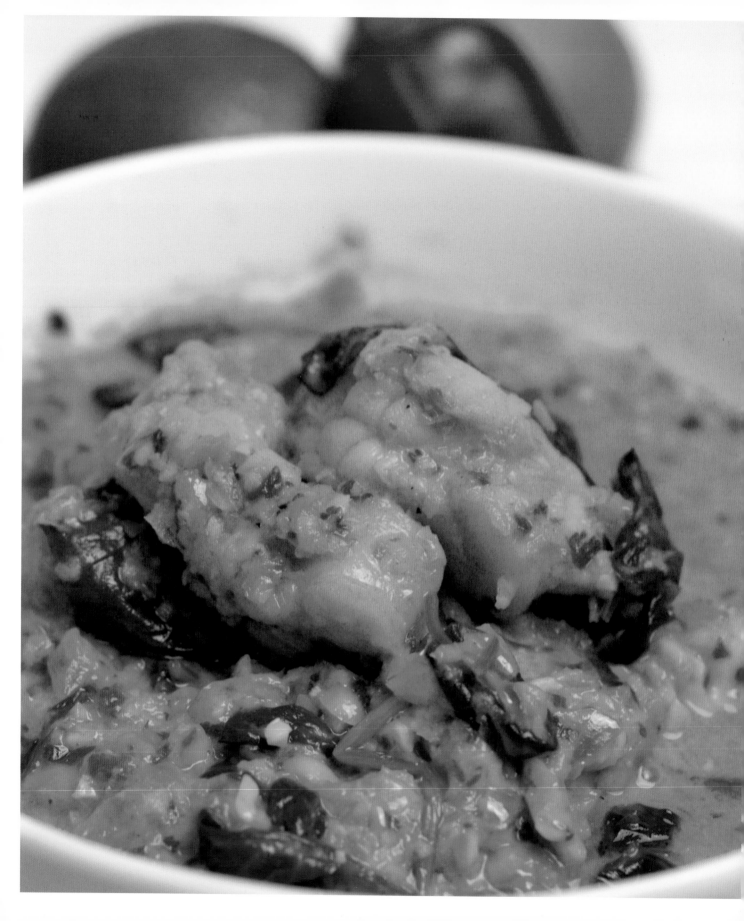

CURRIED MONKFISH WITH SPINACH

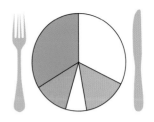

- ■ Fruit & Vegetables
- ☐ Carbohydrates
- ■ Milk, Dairy or Alternatives
- ☐ High in Sugar and/or Fat
- ■ Proteins

This irresistibly flavorful dish is a good example of how to prepare a healthy curry at home without compromising on taste and flavor. While still being creamy, rich and full of flavor, this highly sophisticated dish does not, actually, contain any cream or butter as traditionally curries always do. It's simply made of fresh, easy-to-find ingredients with a balanced blend of spices and herbs. The delicate texture, sweetness and mild flavor of monkfish blend perfectly well with creamy sweet corn, fresh curry leaves, cilantro, garlic, ginger, red chilies and ground turmeric. Monkfish is rich in easily digestible proteins and is also a good source of vitamins B6 and B12 and phosphorus and selenium that act as an antioxidant. When cooking for children, add more or less chili, depending on their taste buds and age. This really is one authentic and comforting dish that all the family will enjoy.

Serves: 2
Preparation Time: 15 min
Cooking Time: 25 min

1 tbsp olive oil
300 g (10.5 oz) monkfish fillet
2 shallots
3 garlic cloves
1 red chili, deseeded
100 g (3.5 oz) frozen sweet corn
2 tbsp fresh cilantro (coriander)
1 tsp ground turmeric
1 tbsp lime juice
100 ml (3.5 fl oz) vegetable stock
100 g (3.5 oz) spinach
200 ml (7 fl oz) light coconut milk
1 tsp grated fresh ginger
2 fresh curry leaves
Salt and freshly ground black pepper

1. Place the shallots, garlic, red chili, sweet corn and cilantro in a small food processor and finely blend to obtain a thick and rich paste.
2. Cut the monkfish fillets into 2 cm (¾ inch) slices, dry with the paper kitchen towel and put aside.
3. Heat the olive oil in a large non-stick frying pan, add grated fresh ginger and curry leaves, stir in the monkfish chunks, and gently fry until lightly browned on all sides.
4. Add the blended mixture, ground turmeric and lime juice into the pan and fry for a further 5 minutes to combine all the flavors.
5. Add the vegetable stock, spinach and coconut milk, season with salt and pepper and bring to the boil, reduce the heat and simmer for 15 minutes or until the sauce becomes thick and smooth.
6. Serve with steamed rice or quinoa.

SPAGHETTI WITH TUNA AND PANGRATTATO

Pasta is such a versatile dish and is one that you hardly ever get bored with. Or at least, this is what we think in Casa Farina – in fact, in Italy this is a 'must have' dish that is usually served as 'Il Primo' a course that is eaten between a starter and a main dish. Even if you cook the same pasta over and over again, you can always dress it up with a different sauce or you can bake it instead, so that you never actually feel that you are having the same dish. It is easy and quick to make, rich in flavor and packed with nutrients. I like to use gluten free brown rice pasta; it is made of the whole grains rather than wheat, is very flavorful and blends well with the sauces. Brown rice pasta is an excellent source of fiber, manganese and energizing B vitamins while canned tuna is rich in proteins and selenium. This tasty dish is an excellent energy booster and a definite winner every time. To add even more flavor to it, always generously sprinkle with Pangrattato (see page 46) to get that Parmesan-like flavor of the dish. Many times good things don't need to be too complicated. Buon appetito!

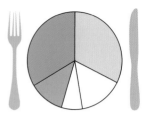

- ■ Fruit & Vegetables
- □ Carbohydrates
- □ Milk, Dairy or Alternatives
- □ High in Sugar and/or Fat
- ■ Proteins

Serves: 4
Preparation Time: 15 min
Cooking Time: 15 min

....

500 g (1 lb 2 oz) GF brown rice spaghetti or any other GF pasta of your choice
2 tbsp olive oil
1 red onion, finely chopped
400 g (14 oz) tuna steak in olive oil
2 garlic cloves, finely chopped
1 red chili, finely chopped
4 tbsp tomato sauce
4 tbsp water, from the cooking pasta
50 g (2 oz) Pangratto (see page 46 for recipe)
Salt and pepper

1. In a large casserole pan, bring 2 liters (4 pints) of water to a boil, add spaghetti and one teaspoon of salt and cook according to the instructions on the packet.
2. In a large non-stick frying pan, heat the olive oil on a medium heat, add chopped onions and gently fry for 2–3 minutes or until golden brown.
3. Stir in the tuna and break the big chunks with a fork.
4. Add the finely chopped garlic and chilies, tomato sauce and a couple of large cooking spoons of hot water (water from the casserole where the pasta is being cooked), mix well, and cook for 5 minutes, stirring occasionally.
5. Transfer the spaghetti from the boiling water just before it is cooked (2 minutes before the end of cooking time) into the mixture and stir for a couple of minutes or until the sauce is evenly mixed with the pasta.
6. Sprinkle generously with pangrattato and serve immediately.

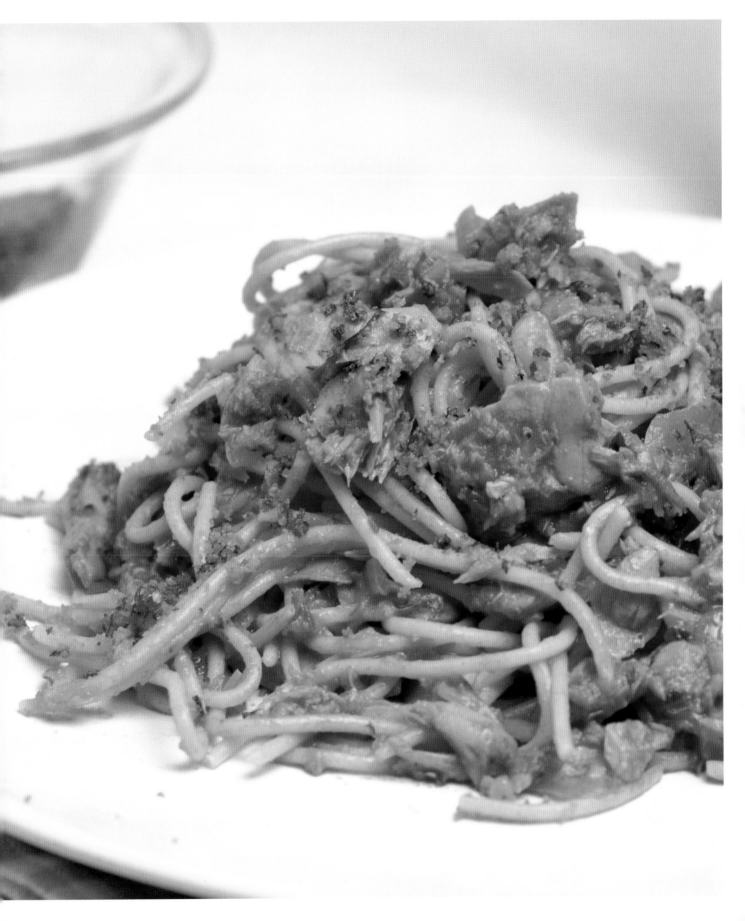

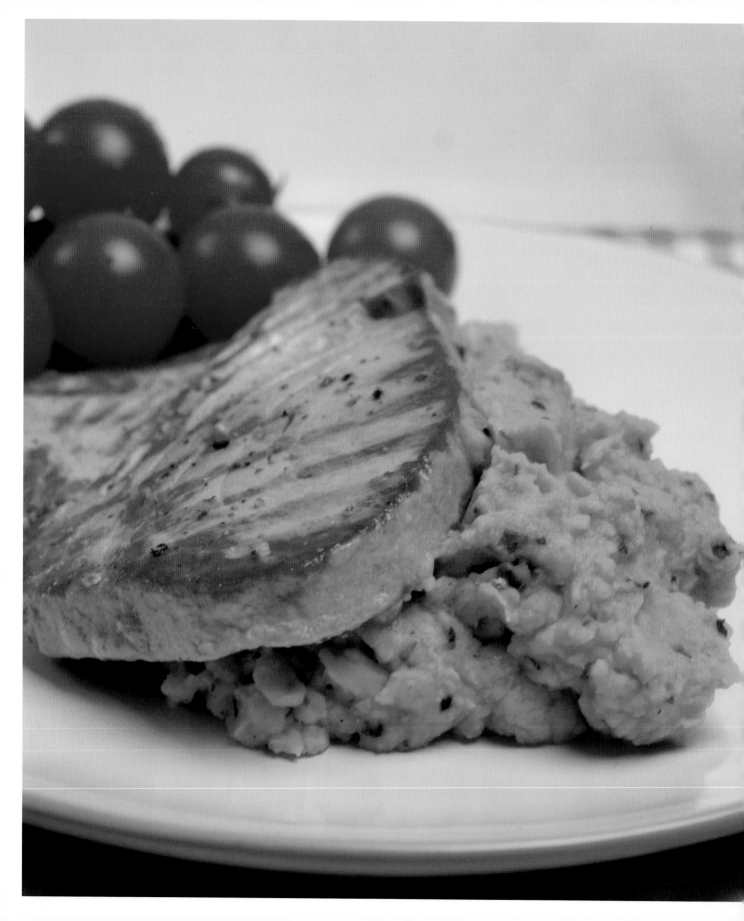

GRILLED TUNA STEAK WITH WHITE BEANS AND CHICKPEA MASH

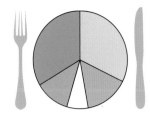

■ Fruit & Vegetables
□ Carbohydrates
■ Milk, Dairy or Alternatives
□ High in Sugar and/or Fat
■ Proteins

I love to make this dish with a grilled tuna steak as long as the tuna is from a non-endangered species. If you cannot find any, it also works a treat with a grilled organic salmon steak. Tuna is naturally rich in omega-3 fatty acids and is also packed with selenium, which has proved beneficial for the health of the skin as an anti-inflammatory. On the other hand, the flavorsome and creamy chickpeas and butter beans combination is a healthy source of dietary fiber, proteins and key vitamins and minerals. Chickpeas are rich in folate, copper and manganese while butter beans are a good source of iron and potassium. This dish is a healthy spin-off from fish and chips in Casa Farina. It's nutrient-packed and a big hit with the children too. OK now, roll up your sleeves and let's get cooking.

Serves: 4
Preparation Time: 5 min
Cooking Time: 15 min

．．

4 tuna steaks (100 g/3.5 oz to 150 g/5 oz each) from a non-endangered species
2 tbsp olive oil
400 g (14 oz) white beans, canned (butter beans or, alternatively, cannellini)
200 g (7 oz) chickpeas, canned
20 ml (0.75 fl oz) water
2 garlic cloves, crushed
50 ml (1.75 fl oz) coconut milk
1 tbsp fresh parsley, finely chopped
1 tbsp fresh basil, finely chopped
Salt and freshly ground black pepper

1. Put the butter beans and chickpeas into a colander and rinse thoroughly with cold water.
2. In a large non-stick frying pan, heat the olive oil on a low heat, add the beans, chickpeas and water and cook for 5 minutes.
3. Add the crushed garlic and mix well.
4. Pour the mixture in a food processor/blender, add the coconut milk, season with salt and pepper and process until your preferred consistency is achieved. Process longer for a smoother consistency. More liquid (coconut milk or water) can be added in the blender if the mixture is too dry.
5. Place the mixture into a large bowl, add the chopped parsley and basil and mix well.
6. In the meantime, grill the tuna steaks in a large grilling pan, 2 minutes on each side. Season with salt and pepper.
7. Serve immediately, placing the tuna steak on top of the beans and chickpea mash.

POACHED COD WITH SWEET PEAS PUREE

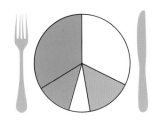

- ▣ Fruit & Vegetables
- ☐ Carbohydrates
- ▣ Milk, Dairy or Alternatives
- ☐ High in Sugar and/or Fat
- ▣ Proteins

Delicious, light and simple, this poached cod and sweet peas dish is packed with proteins and protective phytonutrients. Puree of green peas, having a starchy texture and being sweet in taste, is a delicious and healthy alternative to regular mash potatoes. This dish is guaranteed to be a hit with the whole family. In fact, in Casa Farina, we all love it. It's very tasty, easy and quick to prepare as well as pleasing to the eye due to its bright colors. So, what is there really to complain about?

. . . .

1 tbsp olive oil
400 g (14 oz) cod fillet
50 ml (1.75 fl oz) coconut milk
2 tbsp fresh cilantro (coriander)
1 tsp dry oregano
1 stick lemon grass
300 g (10.5 oz) frozen sweet peas
1 tbsp fresh basil
*Pinch of salt and freshly ground
    black pepper*

Serves: 2
Preparation Time: 10 min
Cooking Time: 15 min

1. Place the cod in a medium pan in a single layer.
2. Add the coconut milk, cilantro, oregano and lemon grass stick and gently bring to boil.
3. Reduce the heat to medium-low, cover and simmer for 10 minutes or until the fish flakes when tested with a fork. Remove from the heat and keep covered.
4. Meanwhile, place the frozen peas in a large saucepan, cover with water and gently bring to boil. Cover and simmer for 5 minutes until cooked. Transfer the peas into a blender, add basil and olive oil and blend until you obtain a smooth and creamy puree.
5. Place the puree on a warm plate and top with a deliciously poached cod fillet.
6. Serve warm.

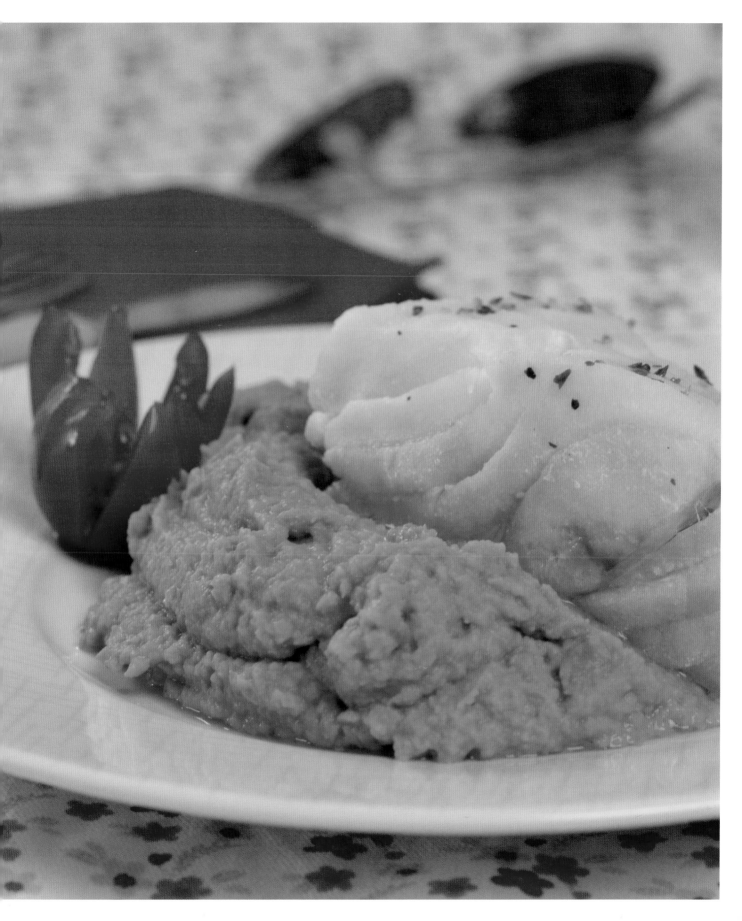

SEAFOOD FRESH TAGLIATELLE

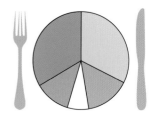

- ■ Fruit & Vegetables
- □ Carbohydrates
- ■ Milk, Dairy or Alternatives
- □ High in Sugar and/or Fat
- ■ Proteins

An all-time Casa Farina favorite, this satisfying and easy to make pasta dish is rich in antioxidants, proteins, omega-3 fatty acids, C vitamins and other nutrients and, above all, is packed with tons of flavor.

The combination of fresh seafood, homemade tomato sauce and coconut cream works perfectly well to create an indulgent thick and creamy seafood sauce that cling incredibly well to the tagliatelle.

This dish is just simply irresistible and will appeal to palates of all ages.

Serves: 4
Preparation Time: 10 min
Cooking Time: 15 min

2 tbsp olive oil
3 garlic cloves, finely chopped
½ red onion, finely chopped
100 g (3.5 oz) smoked salmon, finely chopped
250 g (9 oz) salmon fillet, cut into chunks
150 g (5 oz) raw peeled king shrimp (prawns) tails (whole)
½ red sweet chili
1 tbsp fresh basil, finely chopped
300 ml (10.5 fl oz) tomato sauce (use any readymade GF and DF tomato sauce – or see page 45)
150 ml (5 fl oz) coconut cream
500 g (1 lb 2 oz) fresh GF tagliatelle
Salt and freshly ground black pepper to taste

1. Heat olive oil in a casserole-type saucepan on a medium heat, add chopped garlic and onions and gently fry on a low heat for about 2 minutes or until soft and golden brown.
2. Add smoked salmon, salmon fillet, raw shrimp tails, chopped sweet chilies and basil, season with salt and pepper and cook for 5 minutes, stirring occasionally.
3. Add tomato sauce and coconut cream, mix thoroughly and simmer for 5 minutes, stirring occasionally until you obtain a thick and smooth consistency.
4. In a separate saucepan, bring lightly salted water to the boil, add fresh tagliatelle (see page 41) and cook for 3–4 minutes or until "al dente" (a bit firm but never too soft and overcooked). Follow cooking instructions on the packet if you are using a readymade pasta instead.
5. Drain off the water using a pasta strainer, add a couple of tablespoons of the seafood sauce into a saucepan and a bit of the boiling water of the pasta, mix gently and serve immediately into serving plate.
6. Add seafood sauce as desired, garnish with finely chopped basil and serve immediately.

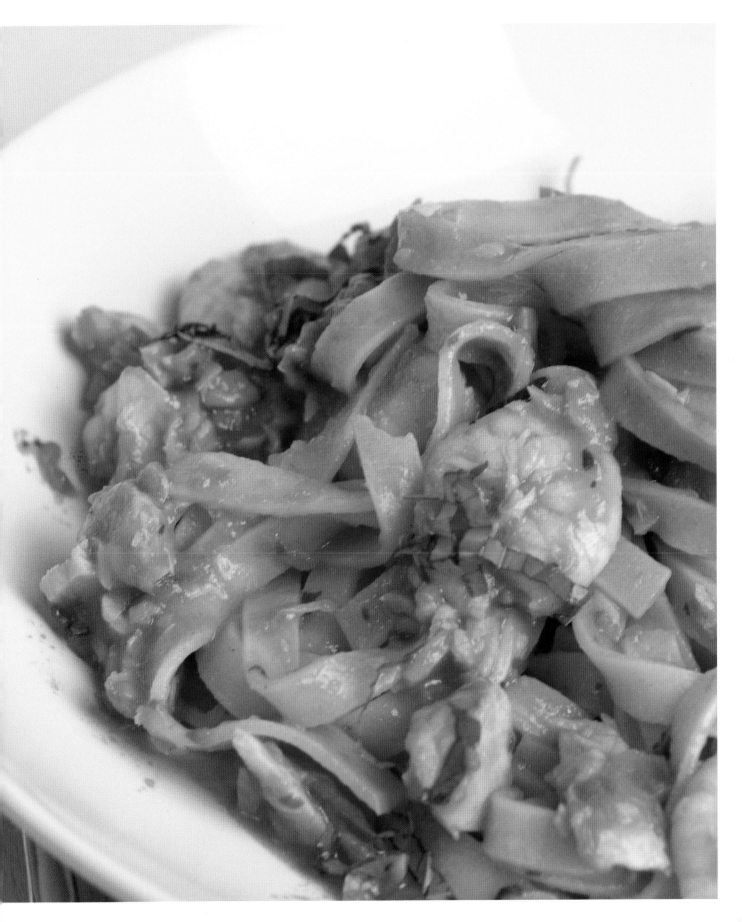

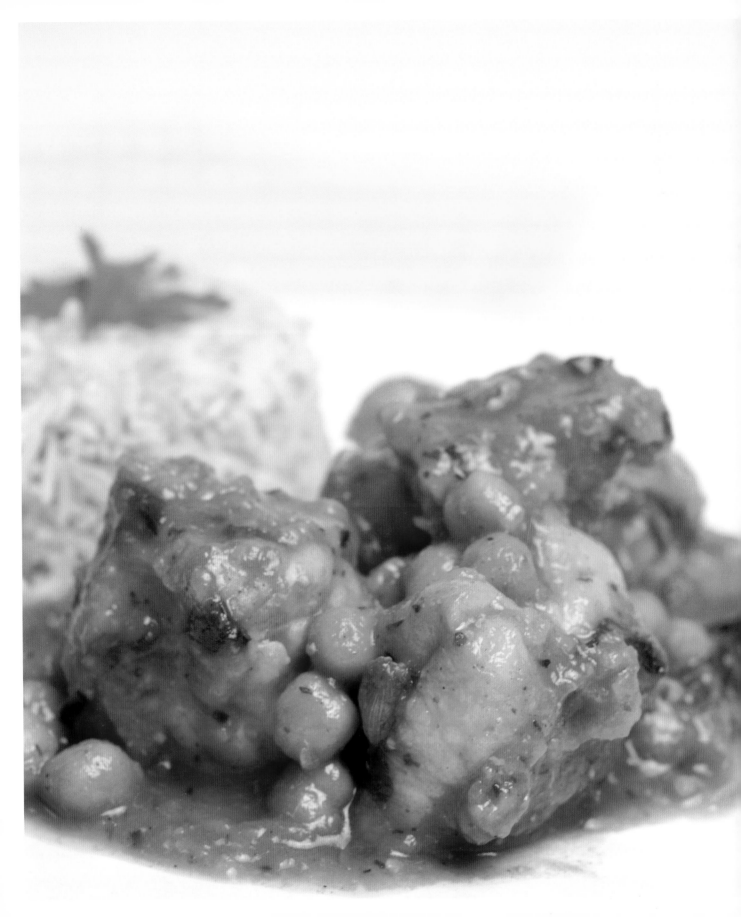

MONKFISH AND CHICKPEAS AMERICANA

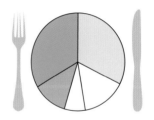

This delightful monkfish and chickpeas combo will satisfy even the fussiest of eaters. The mild and sweet flavor of the monkfish perfectly complements the slightly grainy texture and nutty flavor of the chickpeas. This delicious dish is also packed with masses of nutrients that your body and mind will love. In fact, monkfish naturally contains vitamins B6 and B12 that aid in the synthesis of neurotransmitters needed for brain function. This flavorsome and low fat dish is also rich in easily digestible proteins and dietary fiber.

Serve it warm with rice or quinoa or even with a crunchy salad, and enjoy.

- ▣ Fruit & Vegetables
- ☐ Carbohydrates
- ☐ Milk, Dairy or Alternatives
- ☐ High in Sugar and/or Fat
- ▣ Proteins

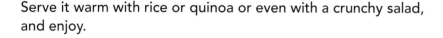

550 g (1 lb 3 oz) monkfish fillet
3 tbsp corn flour
1 tbsp olive oil
3 shallots, finely chopped
4 tbsp tomato paste
400 ml (14 fl oz) vegetable stock
1 tbsp ground paprika
8 cardamom seeds
2 tbsp fresh basil, finely chopped
1 tsp brown sugar
2 tsp anchovy paste
350 g (12 oz) canned chickpeas
*Salt and freshly ground black
    pepper*

Serves: 4
Preparation Time: 20 min
Cooking Time: 25 min

1. Cut the monkfish fillet into large 4 cm (1½ inch) chunks, dry well with kitchen paper and put aside.
2. Place the corn flour into a small bowl and add a pinch of salt. Place each monkfish piece onto the corn flour and gently coat with the flour on all sides, removing any excess flour.
3. Heat the olive oil in a large non-stick frying pan on a medium heat and gently fry the monkfish slices for 5 minutes or until browned on all sides.
4. Add the shallots and gently fry for 3 minutes or until soft. Stir in the tomato paste, vegetable stock, paprika, cardamom seeds, basil, brown sugar, anchovy paste and chickpeas, season with salt and pepper and simmer gently for 15 minutes.
5. Serve warm with steamed rice.

SQUID AND POTATOES STEW

This delightful stew is packed with brilliant flavors and essential nutrients. Soft and slightly sweet squids are a good source of easily digestible proteins, B12 vitamins (essential for red blood cell production) and selenium, while creamy and rich potatoes are packed with complex carbohydrates that provide plenty of sustained energy and other nutrients. This definitely is Casa Farina's favorite stew of all time. Although fresh squids are nowadays readily available, in this recipe, I prefer to use frozen squids as the freezing does not hurt the flavor at all and when slow cooked, it becomes very soft and tender rather than hard and chewy. It's best served warm with a vibrant salad on the side but you can also serve it with boiled rice to make the dish more filling. This stew is definitely a winner every time and at any season. So if you are a seafood lover, go ahead and buy those inexpensive squids and get cooking. Good luck and Buon Appetito!

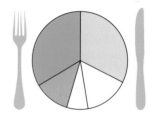

- ▣ Fruit & Vegetables
- ☐ Carbohydrates
- ☐ Milk, Dairy or Alternatives
- ☐ High in Sugar and/or Fat
- ▣ Proteins

Serves: 4
Preparation Time: 15 min
Cooking Time: 60 min

1 tbsp olive oil
5 shallots, finely chopped
1 handful of basil, finely chopped
1 red chili, finely chopped
500 g (1 lb 2 oz) frozen squid tubes,
   defrosted and cut into rings
2 tbsp tomato puree
1 tsp anchovy paste
5 garlic cloves, crushed
1 tsp fish sauce
1 tbsp red Martini
300 g (10.5 oz) white potatoes,
   thick chunks
400 ml (14 fl oz) tomato passata
500 ml (17 fl oz) vegetable stock
1 tsp paprika
1 tbsp parsley, finely chopped
Salt and freshly ground black pepper

1. In a casserole pan, heat the olive oil on a medium heat and gently fry the chopped shallots, basil, and chili for 3 minutes.
2. Stir in the squid, tomato puree, anchovy paste, crushed garlic, fish sauce and red Martini, mix well and continue cooking for a further 3 minutes.
3. Add the potatoes, tomato passata, vegetable stock and season with paprika, salt and pepper. Cover and cook for 40 minutes on a medium heat, stirring occasionally. Remove the cover and cook for a further 20 minutes until the sauce is reduced (thickened) and smooth.
4. Garnish with the chopped parsley. Serve warm.

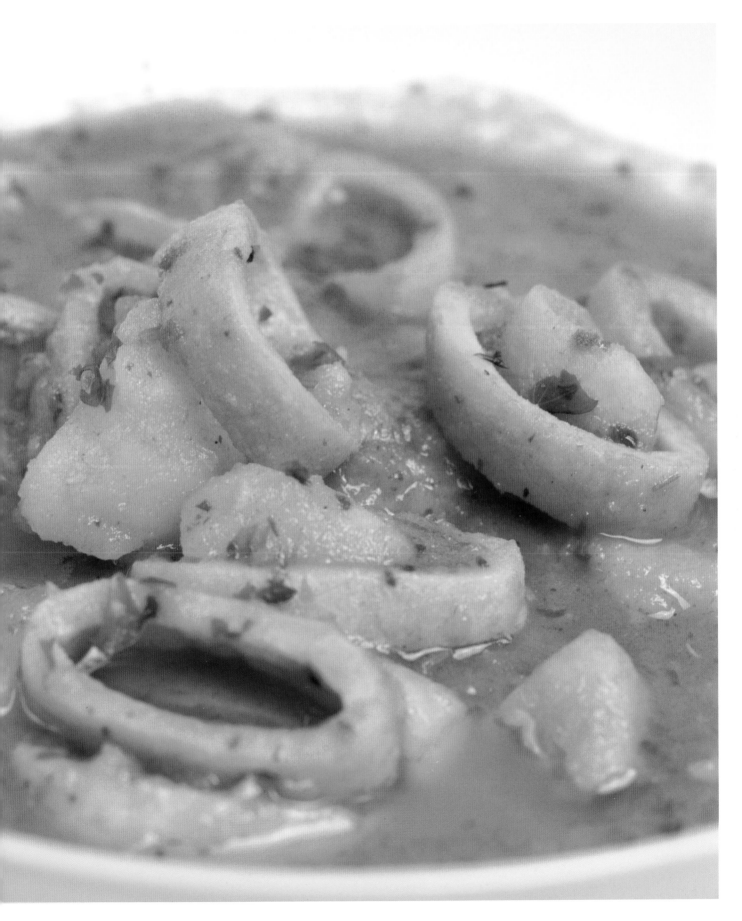

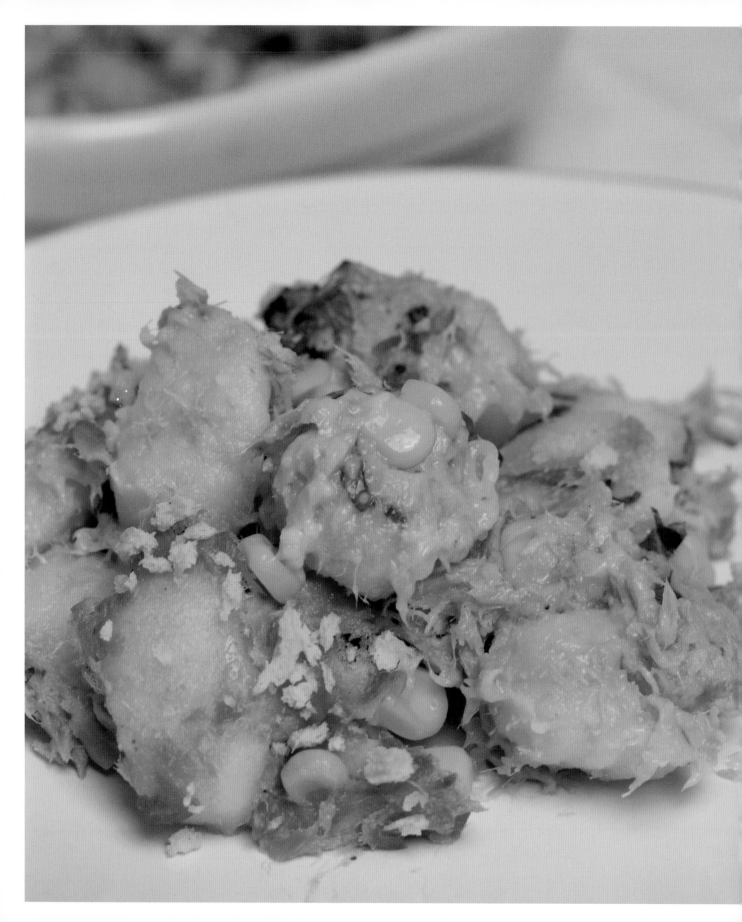

TUNA AND SWEET CORN GNOCCHI BAKE

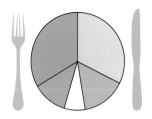

□ Fruit & Vegetables
□ Carbohydrates
□ Milk, Dairy or Alternatives
□ High in Sugar and/or Fat
□ Proteins

This is a healthy alternative to classic tuna and sweet corn pasta bake that is, usually, laden with cheese. Here, I use small potato dumplings, which are naturally gluten free, instead of wheat pasta and, coconut milk, instead of cheese, which is much lighter yet creamy enough to make this dish rich and moist. Tuna is a very good source of protein and is naturally rich in energizing B vitamins, phosphorus and selenium while sweet corn is an excellent source of vitamin E, zinc, dietary fiber and antioxidants.

This simple, nutritious and incredibly tasty bake is always a success. Serve it with your favorite salad and perhaps, a glass of rose. Relax and enjoy.

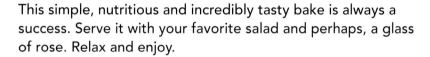

500 g (1 lb 2 oz) potato gnocchi
1 tbsp olive oil
500 ml (17 fl oz) coconut milk
3 tbsp corn flour
20 g (0.75 oz) coconut oil, melted
250 g (9 oz) canned tuna in olive oil, well drained
1 handful of fresh basil, finely chopped
200 g (7 oz) canned sweet corn, drained
GF breadcrumbs or pangrattato
Salt and freshly ground black pepper to taste

Serves: 6
Preparation Time: 10 min
Cooking Time: 35 min

1. Preheat oven to 190°C (375°F).
2. Cook gnocchi in boiling and slightly salty water for 2–3 minutes or until they rise to the surface. (If you are making gnocchi from scratch, see recipe on page 43 but if you are using a shop bought gnocchi, always follow cooking instructions on the pack).
3. Once ready, drain the water off, season with olive oil and keep aside.
4. Pour 50 ml (2 fl oz) of coconut milk into a medium size saucepan, add the corn flour and coconut oil and mix well.
5. Pour the rest of the milk into the saucepan, season with salt and pepper and gently bring to the boil, mixing constantly until the sauce thickens. Remove from heat and keep aside.
6. In a large bowl, add tuna, finely chopped basil and sweet corn, mix well. Pour the milk mixture, add cooked gnocchi and mix thoroughly.
7. Spoon the mixture into a baking tray, generously sprinkle with GF breadcrumbs or pangrattato (see page 46) and bake for 30 minutes or until crispy and golden.
8. Serve warm with your favorite salad.

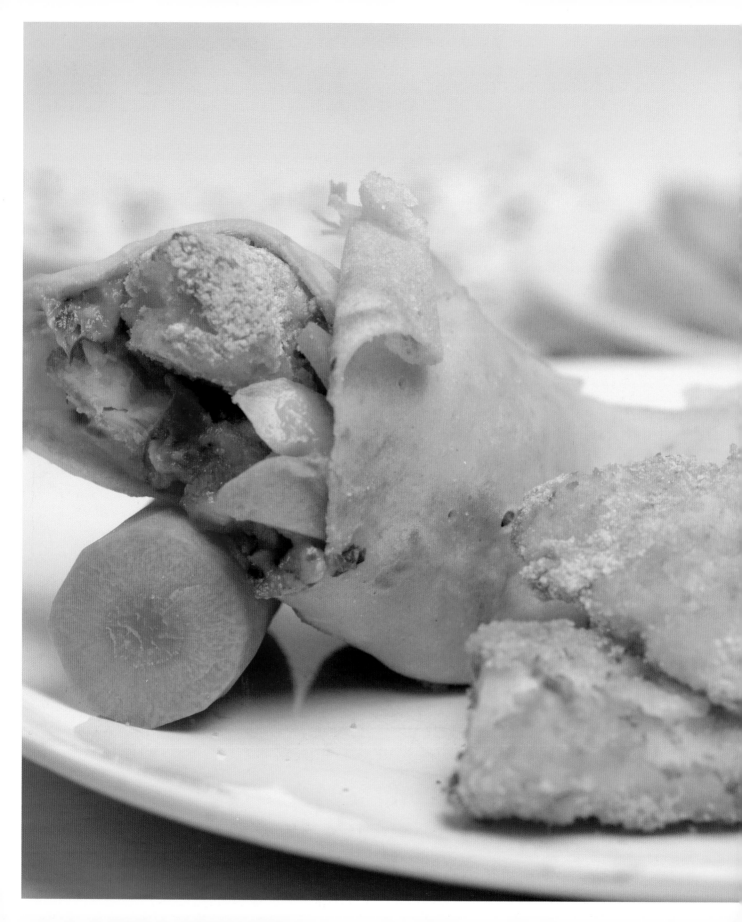

BAKED FISH FINGER PANCAKE WRAPS

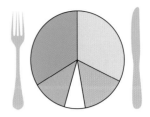

These crisp-baked fish bites are a healthy and nutritious alternative to processed, battered and deep fried fish fingers that we nowadays buy in supermarkets. When combined with fresh julienned carrots and cucumbers (use organic produce whenever possible) and delicious guacamole and then firmly wrapped with a homemade gluten free pancake, they are bound to be a big hit with all, young and old. Traditionally, fish fingers are put into a sandwich and eaten with lots of ketchup and mayonnaise but here I have decided to take more of a healthy route and combine two of my kids big loves: fish fingers and pancakes and make it as healthy and nutritionally balanced as possible. Cod or any other white fish that you decide to use is rich in low fat protein and energizing B vitamins while carrots and cucumber are a good source of vitamins A and C. And after all, who said that the fish fingers fall under the 'junk food' umbrella?

- ☐ Fruit & Vegetables
- ☐ Carbohydrates
- ☐ Milk, Dairy or Alternatives
- ☐ High in Sugar and/or Fat
- ☐ Proteins

400 g (14 oz) cod fillet, thickly sliced
80 g (3 oz) GF breadcrumbs
50 g (1.75 oz) corn meal
1 egg
GF pancakes (see page 49)
1 carrot, julienned
Guacamole (see page 44)
Salt

Serves: 4
Preparation Time: 10 min
Cooking Time: 25 min

1. Preheat oven to 200°C (400°F).
2. Cut the cod fillet into large 2 cm (¾ inch) chunks or finger-length pieces.
3. Place the GF breadcrumbs and corn maize into a large bowl, season with salt and mix well.
4. In a separate small bowl, beat the egg and add a pinch of salt. Now dip the fish fingers, one at the time, firstly in egg batter and gently pierce all the chunks with a fork to allow the egg mixture to enter the meat and give it more moisture. This will also help to seal the coating during the cooking process. As soon as you coat one fish slice with egg, transfer it immediately into the corn maize mixture and gently roll ensuring that the fish finger is coated on all sides. Place the coated fingers on a baking tray lined with a non-stick parchment baking paper, and bake for 25 minutes or until golden crisp.
5. To fill a pancake (see pancake recipe on page 49), firstly place 2–3 fingers lengthwise, add fresh julienned carrots and cucumbers, and spread 1–2 tablespoons of fresh guacamole, firmly roll and eat.
6. Serve warm or cold.

137

POACHED SALMON WITH BEETROOT AND SWEET POTATO MASH

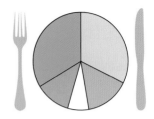

☐ Fruit & Vegetables
☐ Carbohydrates
☐ Milk, Dairy or Alternatives
☐ High in Sugar and/or Fat
☐ Proteins

Serves: 2
Preparation Time: 10 min
Cooking Time: 15 min

I have been experimenting with making a perfect dairy-free mash potato for a long time and this is the recipe that definitely won by far – indulgent and creamy, super healthy and good-looking mash, currently one of my family's favorites. When combined with a protein and omega-3 fats-rich salmon; this really is a wonderfully delicious and simple dish for any occasion. Not only does it taste heavenly, it is very healthy too. Beetroot is a great source of iron and folic acid while sweet potatoes are an excellent energy booster, high in fiber and vitamins A and C. Now, this is a call for all purple color lovers to go ahead and make this beautiful dish. There won't be any regrets, I promise.

200 g (7 oz) sweet potato, boiled
50 g (1.75 oz) white potato
300 g (10.5 oz) salmon fillet (2 fillets)
100 ml (3.5 fl oz) light coconut milk
100 ml (3.5 fl oz) water
2 tbsp chopped chives
2 tbsp olive oil
2 shallots, finely chopped
200 g (7 oz) cooked beetroot in juice, sliced
1 garlic clove, finely chopped
1 tbsp balsamic vinegar
2 tbsp coconut cream
1 tbsp balsamic vinegar glaze (to decorate)
Salt and freshly ground black pepper to taste

1. Peel the white and sweet potatoes, cut them into large chunks and boil for about 10 minutes (or until soft) in a slightly salty water.
2. When the potatoes are cooked, drain off the water, return the potatoes to the saucepan and cover.
3. To poach salmon, place the salmon fillets in a saucepan, add coconut milk (light), water, salt, pepper and 1 tablespoon of finely chopped chives. Bring to a boil, then reduce the heat, cover and simmer for 10 minutes. Remove from the saucepan and set aside to rest until the mash is ready.
4. In a frying pan, add the olive oil, stir in the chopped shallots and gently fry until soft and golden brown. Add the sliced beetroot, chopped garlic, balsamic vinegar, salt and pepper and stir well for about 5 minutes. Add the coconut cream and reduce the consistency to obtain a smooth mixture.
5. Place the mixture into a blender and mash for 30 seconds.
6. Add the boiled potatoes into the blender and blend the mixture again until you obtain a thick, smooth and creamy consistency.
7. To serve, place a large spoon of mash on a plate, add the salmon fillet on top of the mash and sprinkle with chopped chives and olive oil.
8. To decorate, drizzle the balsamic vinegar glaze around the salmon and mash. Enjoy!

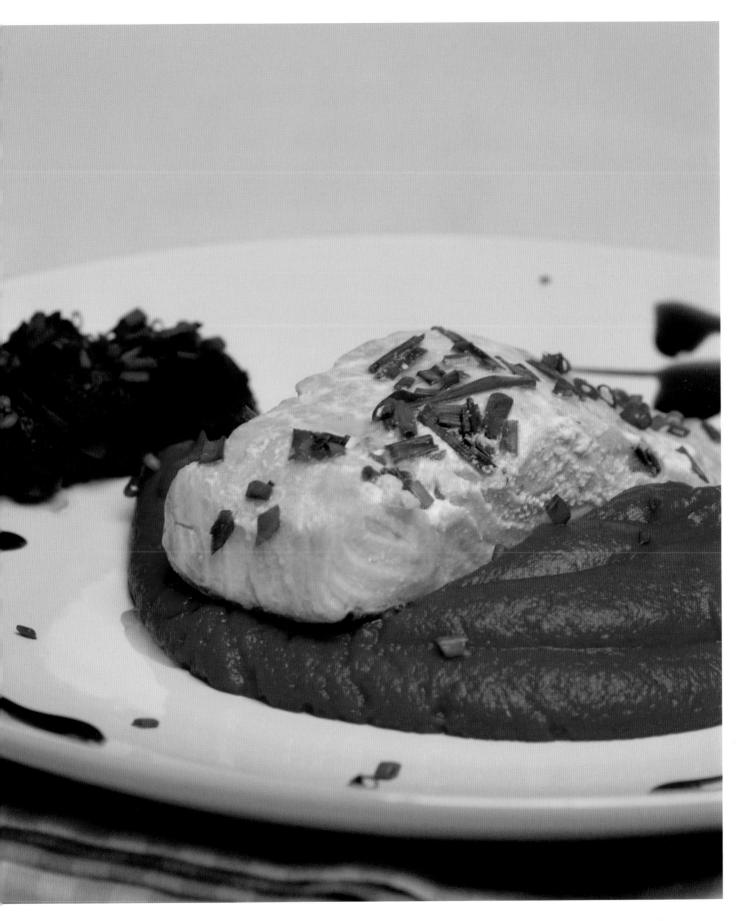

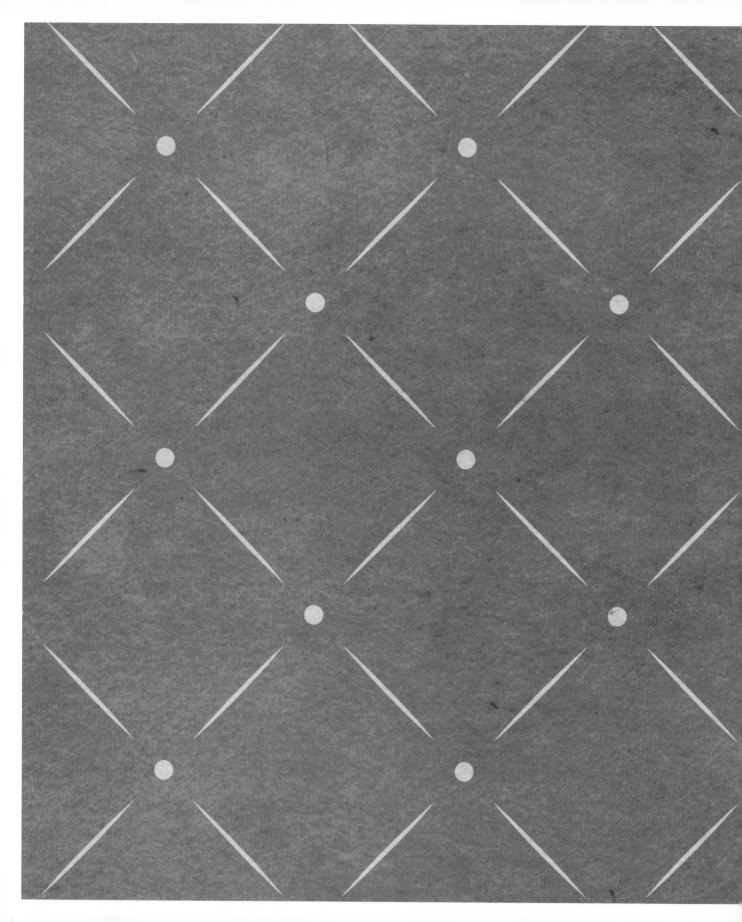

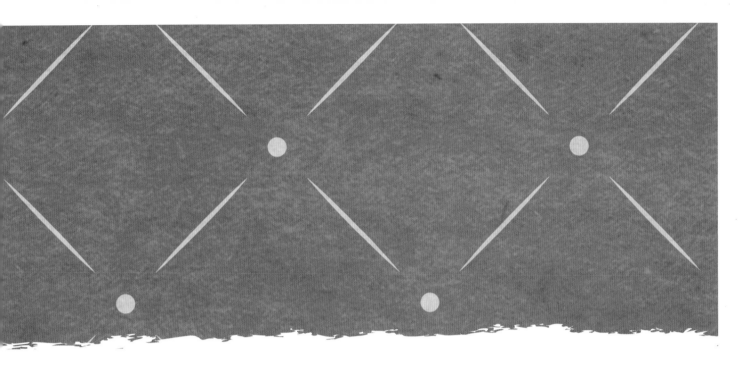

MAINS

·······································

Vegetarian

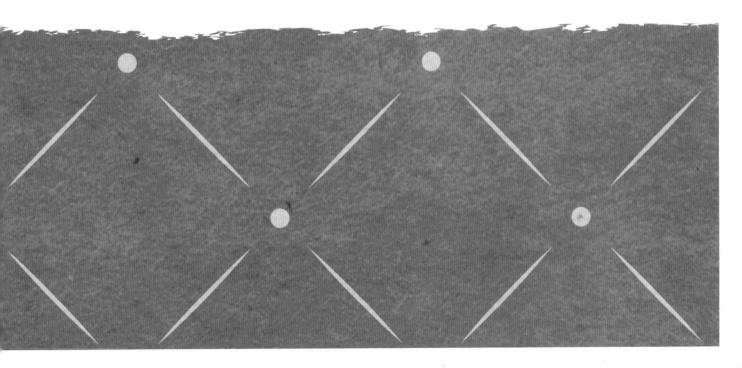

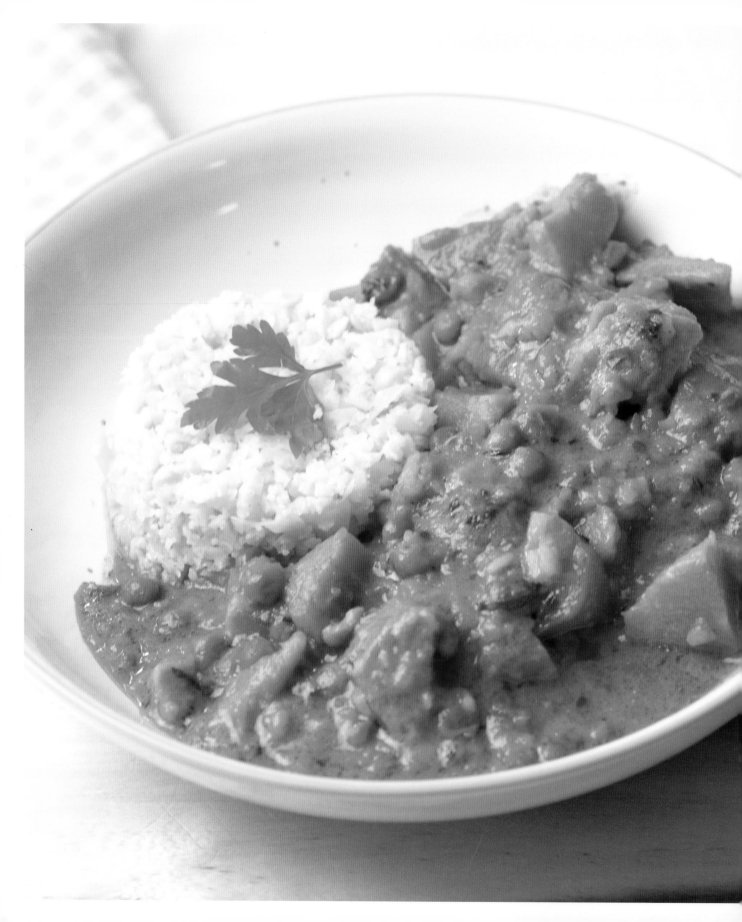

SWEET POTATO CURRY AND CAULIFLOWER RICE

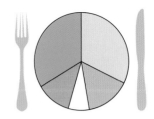

An aromatic blend of delicate spices makes this dish deliciously flavorsome as well as comforting, with a lovely Asian vibe going on. This dish has a mild taste but you may want to add a little bit of fresh chili for your older children. As a healthy alternative to rice, I like to serve it with a super nutritious cauliflower rice instead. This is one of my family's favorite dishes on those rainy days in. Packed with nutrients, wonderfully delicious and full of flavor – what is there to complain about?

☑ Fruit & Vegetables
☐ Carbohydrates
☑ Milk, Dairy or Alternatives
☐ High in Sugar and/or Fat
☑ Proteins

Sweet Potato Curry

1 tbsp olive oil
1 red onion, chopped
1 tbsp tomato puree
½ tsp sweet paprika
A pinch of cardamom
A pinch of cumin
½ tsp turmeric
1 tsp fresh ginger, grated
1 garlic clove, crushed
A pinch of salt
150 g (5 oz) frozen peas
4 sweet potatoes, cubed
1 carrot, peeled and cubed
1 zucchini (courgette), cubed
1 can of coconut milk

Cauliflower Rice

250 g (9 oz) cauliflower florets
1 tbsp olive oil
A pinch of salt

Serves: 6
Preparation Time: 15 min
Cooking Time: 45 min

1. For the Sweet Potato Curry: add one tablespoon of olive oil into a large frying and sauté red onion until soft.
2. Stir in the tomato puree and all spices (paprika, cardamom, cumin, turmeric, ginger, garlic, salt) mixing thoroughly to form a paste. Once the paste is formed, dilute with a little bit of water to obtain a more liquid consistency.
3. Stir in the frozen peas, cubed sweet potatoes, carrots and zucchini and continue to cook for a further 5 minutes. Add the coconut milk and bring the mixture to a rapid simmer, stirring constantly.
4. Reduce the heat and simmer gently for around 40 minutes until all vegetables are soft, adding a little more water if the mixture becomes too dry. Serve warm.
5. For the Cauliflower Rice: place the cauliflower florets into a food blender and blend until you get a texture of rice (do not over process, as the cauliflower can get mushy).
6. Heat one tablespoon of olive oil on a medium heat, stir in the processed cauliflower, add a pinch of salt and sauté for about 5 minutes or until soft, stirring constantly. Add some water if the texture becomes too dry.
7. Serve warm with curry or other dishes.

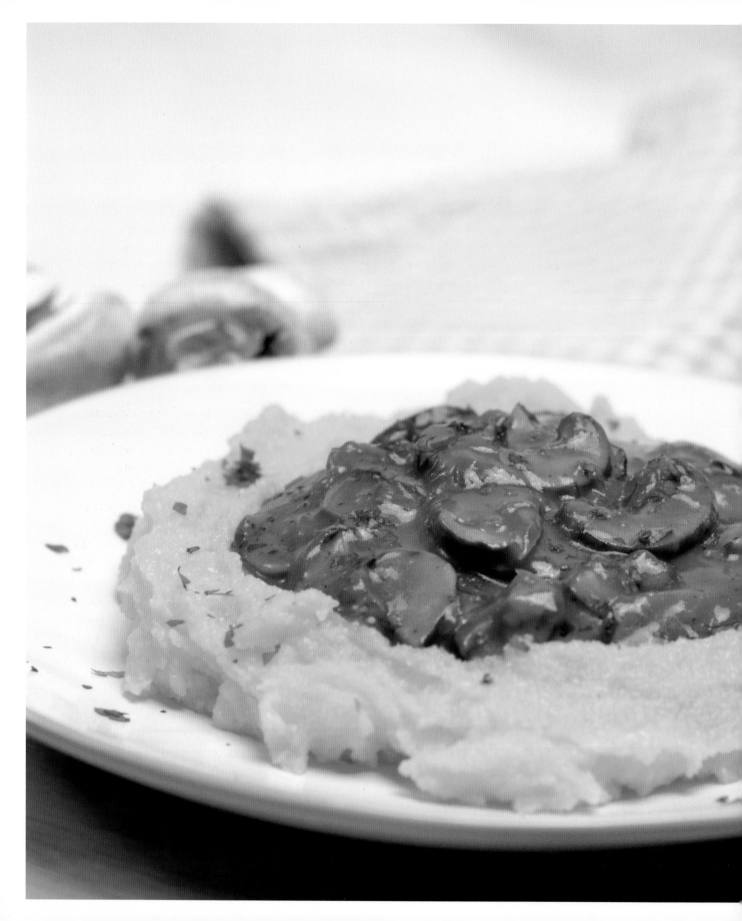

POLENTA WITH CREAMY MUSHROOMS MEDLEY

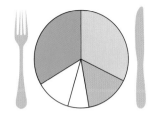

Rich and full of flavor, this creamy polenta dish is best served warm. Polenta is a delicious gluten free alternative to pasta, mashed potatoes or rice and an excellent source of fiber and energizing B vitamins. It's also a good source of slow-releasing carbohydrates making you fuller for longer. On the other hand, mushrooms provide an extra serving of vegetables and are a good source of antioxidants and vitamin D. For all the mushroom lovers, this definitely is a 'must have' super dish.

- ☐ Fruit & Vegetables
- ☐ Carbohydrates
- ☐ Milk, Dairy or Alternatives
- ☐ High in Sugar and/or Fat
- ☐ Proteins

....

2 tbsp olive oil
2 garlic cloves, finely chopped
1 red onion, finely chopped
1 tbsp fresh parsley, finely chopped
1 tbsp tomato paste
450 g (16 oz) mixed fresh mushrooms (chestnut and ceps but can also use others such as chanterelles oysters etc.)
2 tbsp fresh lemon juice
200 ml (7 fl oz) vegetable stock
100 ml (3.5 fl oz) coconut cream
1 tbsp corn flour
2 tbsp water
150 g (5 oz) polenta (boiled in 150 ml (5 fl oz) of lightly salted water)
Salt and freshly ground black pepper to taste

Serves: 6
Preparation Time: 20 min
Cooking Time: 35 min

1. Heat olive oil in a saucepan on a medium heat, add chopped garlic, onion and a half tablespoon of parsley and gently fry for 2 minutes or until soft and golden brown. Add tomato paste and mix thoroughly.
2. Add the sliced mushrooms and lemon juice and cook for 10 minutes, stirring occasionally.
3. Add the vegetable stock, season with salt and freshly ground black pepper, cover the saucepan and simmer for 15 minutes.
4. In a separate saucepan, bring 150 ml (5 fl oz) of lightly salty water to the boil, add polenta, mix well and cook following the instructions on the packet. (For this recipe I am using quick precooked polenta that only takes 8 minutes to cook). Stir the polenta for 5 minutes, add half a tablespoon of olive oil, remove from the heat and let it simmer.
5. Uncover the mushroom mixture, add the coconut milk and let it simmer for 10 minutes.
6. Mix the corn flour with two tablespoons of water in a small bowl and stir into the mushroom mixture.
7. Reduce the heat, simmer for a further 2–3 minutes, stirring constantly, until the sauce thickens and becomes creamy.
8. Transfer the polenta onto a serving plate, make a wheel in the middle, add the creamy mushrooms medley, sprinkle over the remaining parsley and serve immediately.

SPAGHETTI WITH BASIL PESTO SAUCE

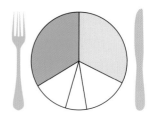

This irresistibly delicious dish is full of nutrients and flavor.
Basil is rich in vitamins, A, C and K and is also a good source
of iron, magnesium and calcium. It's packed with antioxidants
and contains essential oils that help to reduce inflammation
and swelling. Garlic also has antioxidant properties, it's packed
with sulphurous compounds that are responsible for liver
detoxification and immune function and is rich in vitamin C,
vitamin B6 and manganese. This dish is so simple and quick
to make but yet delicious and healthy too. Pangrattato adds
that extra crunchiness while basil, garlic and olive oil blend
beautifully together to give that smooth and rich flavor.
When the time is limited, this dish is always a winner.

■ Fruit & Vegetables
☐ Carbohydrates
☐ Milk, Dairy or Alternatives
☐ High in Sugar and/or Fat
☐ Proteins

400 g (14 oz) GF spaghetti
100 g (3.5 oz) fresh basil leaves
2 garlic cloves
50 ml (1.75 fl oz) olive oil
*40 g (1.5 oz) pangrattato (see
 recipe page 46)*

Serves: 4
Preparation Time: 5 min
Cooking Time: 10 min

1. Fill a deep casserole pan ¾ full with water, add 1 teaspoon of
coarse sea salt for every 2 liters of water, and bring to the boil.
2. Add the spaghetti and cook according to the instructions on the
packet or until "al dente". Taste the pasta regularly to ensure you do
not overcook it. Pour the pasta into a strainer and drain off – keep
some of the water where the pasta was cooked aside.
3. In the meantime, place the basil leaves, garlic and olive oil into
an electric chopper and pulse until fully incorporated smooth and
creamy.
4. Place the sauce into a small bowl, add 30 g (1 oz) of pangrattato,
3 tablespoons of the boiling pasta water and mix well. Place the pasta
into the bowl, add the pesto sauce and 2 tablespoons of the boiling
pasta water and mix well.
5. Serve immediately.

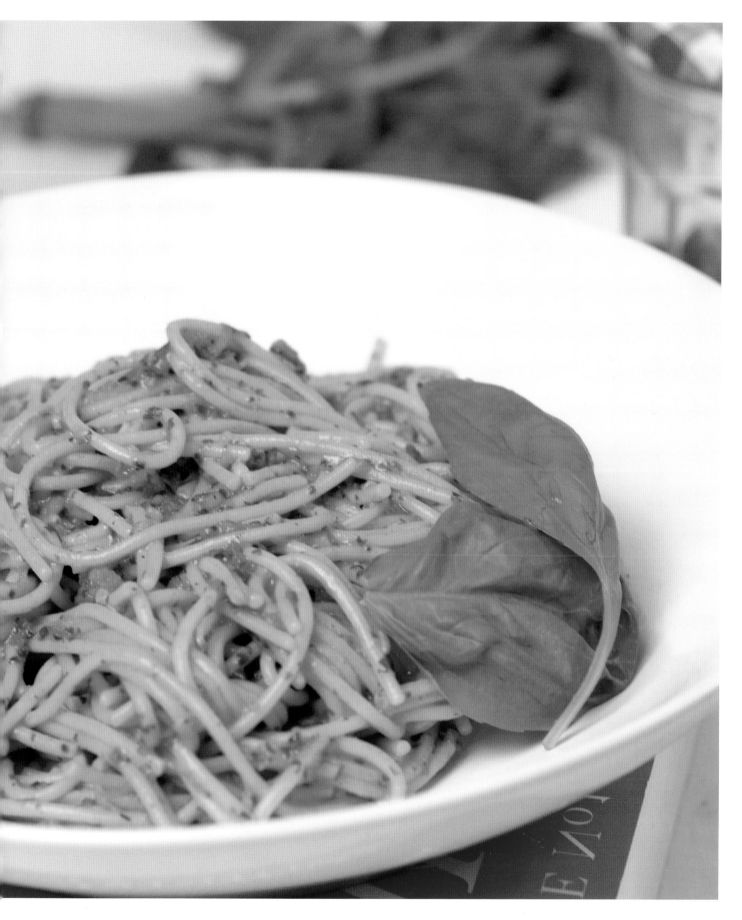

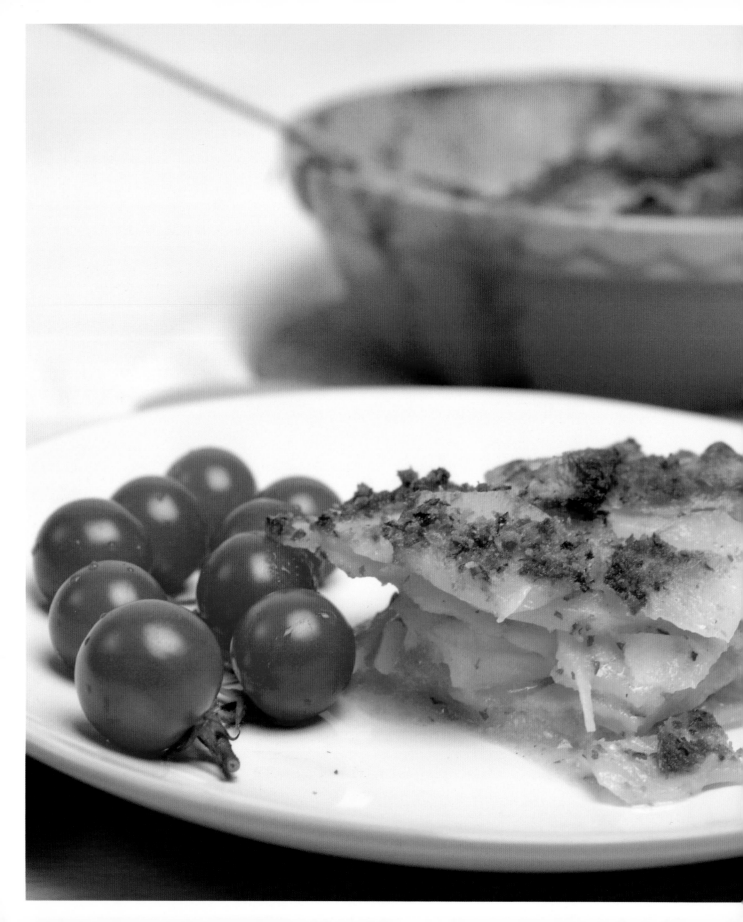

POTATOES AND JERUSALEM ARTICHOKES DAUPHINOISE

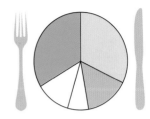

This definitely is the best potatoes dauphinoise I have ever tasted. In my view, this is clearly a step up from traditional gratin dauphinoise where the potatoes are slowly baked with cream and garlic. In this recipe we use a fresh root vegetable tuber called Jerusalem artichokes. The rich, nutty, sweet and strong flavor of this vegetable is just magical and perfectly complements creamy potatoes. Make sure that you don't mistake Jerusalem artichokes with 'normal' globe artichokes as the flavor is very different. Always look for the varieties that are free from spots and sprouting. This delicate flavored root vegetable of the sunflower family (also called sunchoke or sunroot) is rich in soluble fiber, vitamin C, potassium, iron and thiamine. It also complements meat and fish dishes.

- Fruit & Vegetables
- Carbohydrates
- Milk, Dairy or Alternatives
- High in Sugar and/or Fat
- Proteins

Serves: 6
Preparation Time: 15 min
Cooking Time: 60 min

---

500 g (1 lb 2 oz) white potatoes, peeled and thin sliced
300 g (10.5 oz) Jerusalem artichokes, peeled and thinly sliced
100 ml (3.5 fl oz) coconut cream
250 ml (9 fl oz) light coconut milk
1 tsp dried thyme
1 tsp dried oregano
1 garlic clove, crushed
1 tsp cayenne pepper
1 tsp corn flour
2 tbsp olive oil
4 shallots, finely chopped
60 g (2 oz) pangrattato (see recipe page 46)
Salt and freshly ground black pepper

1. Preheat oven to 180°C (350°F).
2. Thinly slice the potatoes and Jerusalem artichokes, place in a medium-size bowl, season with salt and freshly ground black pepper and mix well.
3. Tip the coconut cream, milk, thyme, dried oregano, crushed garlic, cayenne pepper, corn flour, salt and pepper into a saucepan and simmer gently for 5 minutes. Remove from the heat and put aside.
4. Heat the olive oil in a small non-stick frying pan, add the shallots and gently fry for 2–3 minutes or until soft and light brown.
5. Place half of the shallots mixture on the bottom of the 2 liter (2 quart) baking dish, add a layer of sliced potatoes and Jerusalem artichokes mixture and finish with the remaining fried shallots on top of the dish and then sprinkle generously with pangrattato.
6. Pour in the coconut cream and milk mixture.
7. Cover with pangrattato and bake for one hour or until Jerusalem artichokes are soft and cooked through (please note that it takes a bit longer for Jerusalem artichokes to cook).
8. Serve warm on its own or with a crunchy salad on the side.

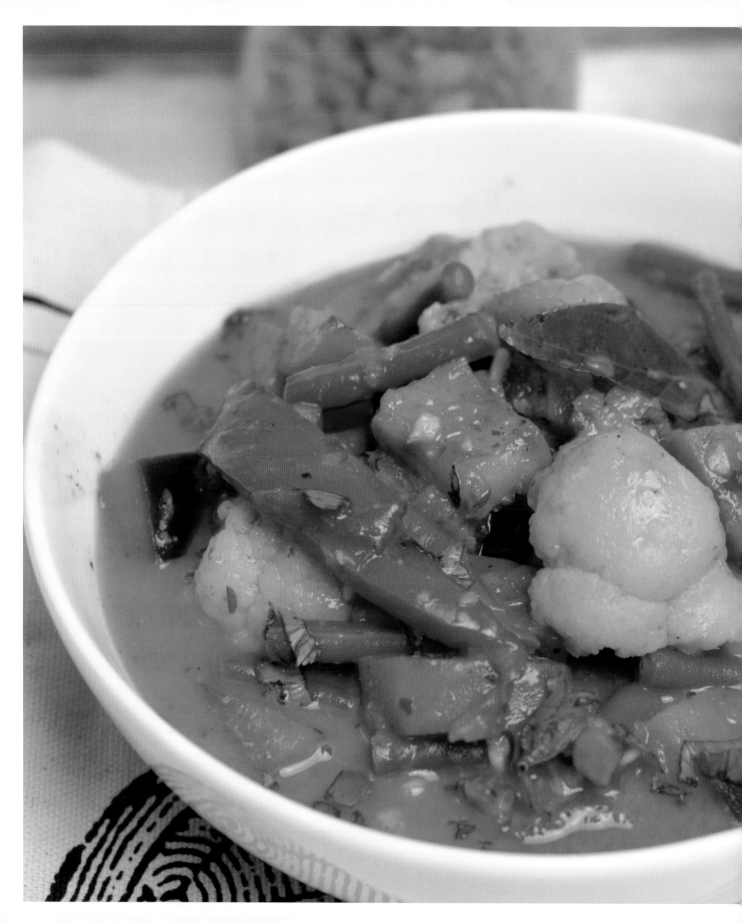

VEGETABLE CURRY

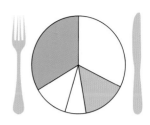

This incredibly flavorful, Asian-inspired dish is a 'must have' vegetarian option for a super healthy main course. With all the aromatic spices and variety of vegetables, this dish is bursting with nutrients and flavor. Add more or less chili depending of your taste buds. This really is a perfect, hearty and comforting dish for those long wintery days.

- ■ Fruit & Vegetables
- ☐ Carbohydrates
- ■ Milk, Dairy or Alternatives
- ☐ High in Sugar and/or Fat
- ☐ Proteins

1 tbsp vegetable oil
1 onion, finely chopped
4 cardamom pods
1 handful of fresh cilantro
   (coriander), finely chopped
1 garlic clove
2 tsp ground cumin
2 tsp ground cilantro (coriander)
1 tsp turmeric
20 g (0.75 oz) fresh root ginger,
   peeled and grated
1 green chili, deseeded and finely
   chopped
400 ml (14 fl oz) vegetable stock
300 ml (10.5 fl oz) coconut milk
450 g (1 lb) mixed vegetables, cut
   into large chunks
Salt

Serves: 4
Preparation Time: 10 min
Cooking Time: 30 min

1. Heat the oil in a large casserole type pan, add finely chopped onions and gently fry until soft and golden. Add the cardamom pods, fresh cilantro, garlic, cumin, ground cilantro, turmeric, ginger, green chili and mix thoroughly to combine the flavors.
2. Pour in the vegetable stock and coconut milk, add diced vegetables, season with salt, cover and cook for 15 minutes or until the vegetables are soft.
3. Uncover and reduce the curry sauce for further 10 minutes.
4. Generously sprinkle with fresh cilantro and serve warm with steamed rice or on its own.

SPINACH AND MUSHROOM CANNELLONI

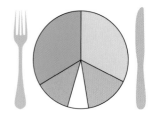

A healthy twist on classic spinach and ricotta cannelloni, this recipe is far lower in fat than traditional cannelloni that is laden with ricotta and mozzarella cheese. This flavorful cannelloni dish is perfect for a healthy vegetarian main course. To make it meaty, simply fill the homemade pancakes or cannelloni tubes with a meat ragu. This delicious dish in packed with plenty of nutrients too. Spinach is rich in antioxidants and is naturally high in iron, vitamin C, vitamin B6 and calcium while chestnut mushrooms are an excellent source of proteins, vitamins B and D and potassium. Hearty and strong in flavor, chestnut mushrooms are a good substitute to meat.

◼ Fruit & Vegetables
☐ Carbohydrates
◼ Milk, Dairy or Alternatives
☐ High in Sugar and/or Fat
◼ Proteins

2 tbsp olive oil
250 g (9 oz) chestnut mushrooms, cleaned and finely chopped
1 garlic clove, crushed
1 tbsp chives, finely chopped
160 g (5.5 oz) fresh spinach
1 egg
2 tbsp coconut cream
5 tbsp brown rice flour
10 homemade pancakes (GF, DF and SF (see recipe page 49) or use 15–20 GF and DF cannelloni tubes)
250 ml (9 fl oz) tomato sauce
Salt and freshly ground black pepper

Serves: 6
Preparation Time: 10 min
Cooking Time: 40 min

1. Preheat oven to 190°C (375°F).
2. In a non-stick frying pan, heat the olive oil on a medium heat, stir in the mushrooms, garlic, chives, season with salt and pepper, mix well and gently fry for 5 minutes.
3. Firmly squash the fresh spinach and with your hands squeeze out the excess water before adding it in the mixture.
4. Add into the mixture and gently fry for 5 minutes or until the spinach leaves have reduced in volume and the juice has evaporated. Remove the mushrooms and spinach mixture from the heat and let it cool down for 5 minutes.
5. Place the mixture into a bowl, add egg, coconut cream, brown rice flour and mix well to form a compact stuffing. Add more flour if the mixture is too liquid.
6. Place 3 tablespoons of the mixture in the center of each pancake and firmly roll to form a cannelloni tube. Lay the cannelloni side by side into a greased baking tray and repeat until you fill the tray. You can now freeze the cannelloni uncooked or cook it first and then freeze.
7. Pour over the tomato sauce until the pasta is covered, leaving only, the edges uncovered so they become crispy and golden brown. Bake for 25 minutes until golden and bubbling.
8. Remove from the oven and let stand for 5 minutes before serving.
9. Serve warm on its own or with a crunchy salad on the side.

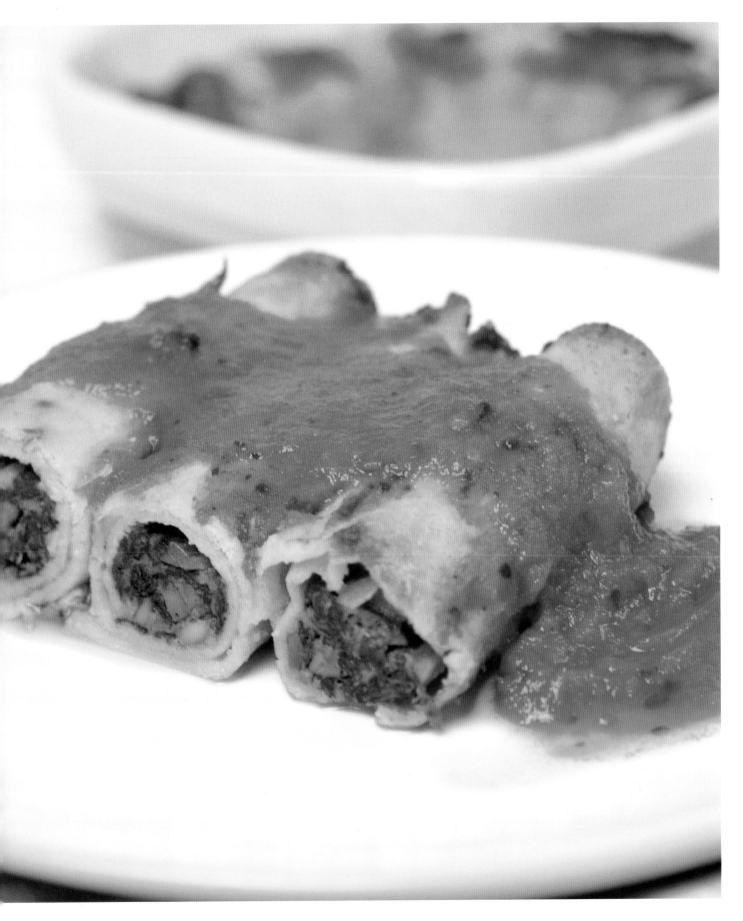

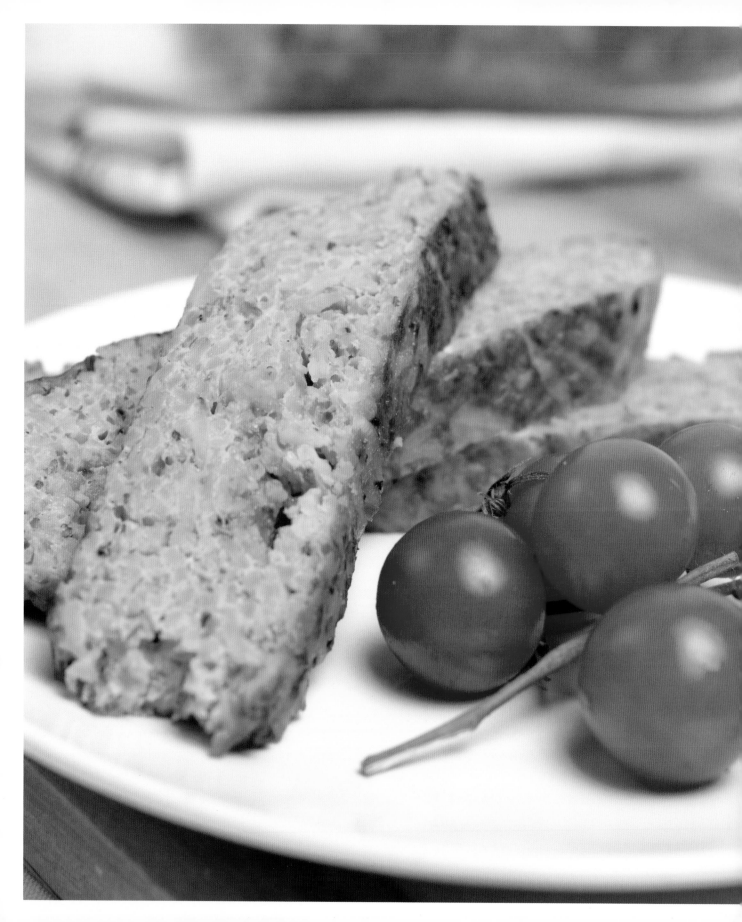

VEGETABLE RICE BAKE

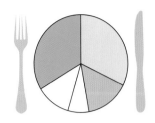

This hearty and comforting rice bake is full of flavor and nutrients. Packed with vegetables, this really is the simplest way of getting zucchinis, broccoli and carrots into your child's diet. You can easily play around with the types and proportions of vegetables used. This bake is also rich in eggs, which are a complete source of protein and packed with vitamin D, selenium, vitamin B12 and iron. This satisfying dish is an all-time family favorite.

- ◼ Fruit & Vegetables
- ◻ Carbohydrates
- ◼ Milk, Dairy or Alternatives
- ◻ High in Sugar and/or Fat
- ◻ Proteins

100 g (3.5 oz) rice (basmati or other)
300 g (10.5 oz) mixed fresh vegetables (carrot, zucchini (courgette) and broccoli)
1 tbsp olive oil
1 onion finely chopped
150 ml (5 fl oz) vegetable stock
100 ml (3.5 fl oz) coconut milk
1 tbsp fresh basil, chopped
½ tsp turmeric powder
1 tbsp chives, finely chopped
3 eggs
Salt and freshly ground black pepper

Serves: 6
Preparation Time: 20 min
Cooking Time: 30 min

1. Preheat oven to 180°C (350°F).
2. Boil rice as per instructions on the packet and keep aside in a large bowl. (Cooking times differ depending on the type of rice used). For this recipe I used basmati rice.
3. Peel and wash the vegetables, place into an electric food processor and finely chop.
4. In a large non-stick frying pan, gently heat the olive oil on a medium heat, add chopped onions and gently fry for 2–3 minutes or until soft and slightly browned.
5. Add chopped vegetables (carrots, zucchini and broccoli), vegetable stock, coconut milk, basil and turmeric. Simmer and keep uncovered for 10 minutes or until the vegetables are soft and the sauce has reduced.
6. Place the mixture into a medium size bowl, add cooked rice, chopped chives, eggs, season with salt and pepper and mix well.
7. Pour the mixture into a greased 1.5 liter (1½ quart) baking dish and bake for 30 minutes.
8. Serve warm.

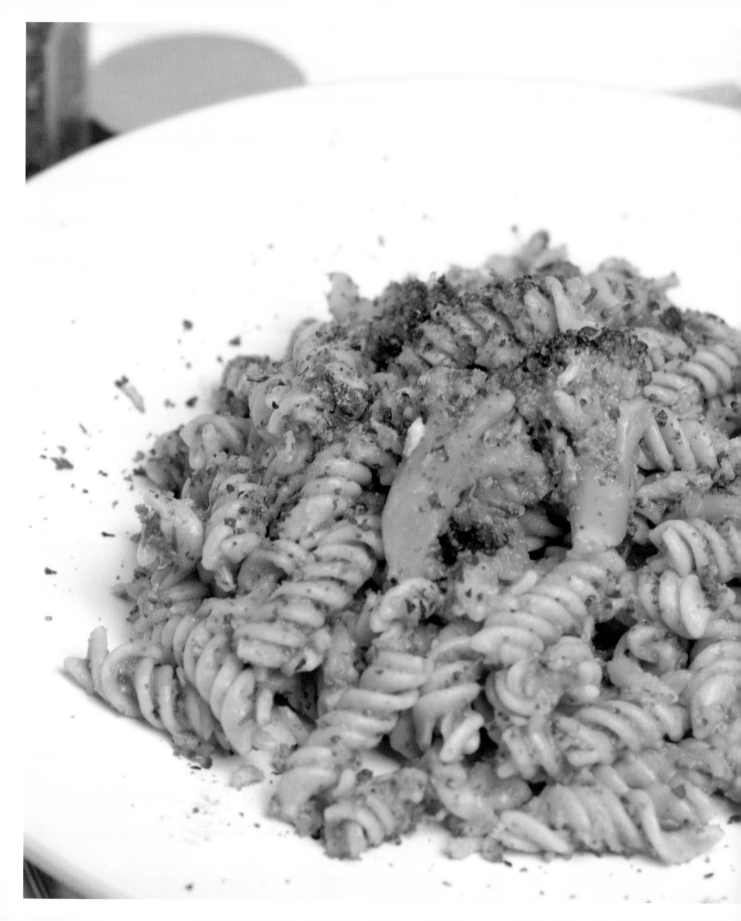

FUSILLI WITH BROCCOLI AND GARLIC

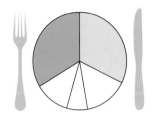

Spaghetti with broccoli and garlic make a comforting, nutritious dish that is simple and speedy to put together. Garlic is rich in vitamin C, vitamin B6 and manganese and also contains trace amounts of various other nutrients. It acts as a natural antibiotic and when consumed, helps to protect against bacterial, parasite and yeast infections. Garlic is also rich in sulphurous compounds that are responsible for liver detoxification and immune function. On the other hand, broccoli is a good source of iron, folic acid and fiber. It is packed with antioxidants that help to protect against cell damage and also have anti-cancer properties. This dish is made in minutes and loved by everyone.

- ▣ Fruit & Vegetables
- ☐ Carbohydrates
- ☐ Milk, Dairy or Alternatives
- ☐ High in Sugar and/or Fat
- ☐ Proteins

2 tbsp olive oil
5 garlic cloves, crushed
100 ml (3.5 fl oz) tomato sauce
300 g (10.5 oz) fresh broccoli florets
400 g (14 oz) GF fusilli (brown rice fusilli)
30 g (1 oz) pangrattato (see recipe page 46)

Serves: 4
Preparation Time: 5 min
Cooking Time: 10 min

1. Heat 2 tablespoons of olive oil in a small saucepan on a low heat. Stir in the crushed garlic and gently fry for only 1 minute to release the flavor and, immediately, pour in the tomato sauce. Do not overcook the garlic. Gently simmer for 5 minutes on a low heat and put aside.
2. In the meantime, fill a deep casserole pan ¾ full with water, add 1 teaspoon of coarse sea salt for every 2 liters of water, and bring to the boil.
3. Add the broccoli florets and cook for 5 minutes until almost soft.
4. Add the spaghetti to the boiling water with broccoli and cook according to the instructions on the packet or until "al dente". Taste the pasta regularly to ensure you do not overcook it.
5. When the pasta is cooked, pour the pasta and broccoli into a pasta strainer and drain off – keep some of the boiling water aside for later use.
6. Place pasta and broccoli into a large bowl, add the garlic and tomato sauce and 2 tablespoons of pasta water to loosen and mix well. The broccoli will break down and form a creamy sauce. Add more water if the sauce is too dry.
7. Sprinkle with pangrattato and serve immediately.

FRESH PASTA FRITTATA

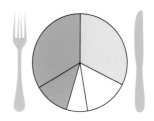

This is quick, easy and yet a wonderfully tasty dish that all family will enjoy. It's also a perfect way to use up all your pasta leftovers. It is rich in eggs, which are a complete source of high quality proteins and B12 vitamin which is vital for the nervous system and development of red blood cells. They are also an important source of zinc, iron, selenium and other energizing B vitamins. This incredibly simple, energizing and brain-boosting dish is a perfect lunch choice for the whole family. In order to help the absorption of iron, it is beneficial to combine this dish with a citrusy salad rich in vitamin C. In Casa Farina we love to eat Pasta Frittata just before we go for a long walk in the park. It gives you energy to walk for a long time before you get hungry again.

■ Fruit & Vegetables
☐ Carbohydrates
☐ Milk, Dairy or Alternatives
☐ High in Sugar and/or Fat
■ Proteins

---

400 g (14 oz) fresh GF pasta
1 tbsp olive oil
3 tbsp tomato sauce
5 eggs
Salt and freshly ground black
* pepper*

Serves: 4
Preparation Time: 5 min
Cooking Time: 10 min

1. Cook 400 g (14 oz) of fresh GF pasta (see page 41) or (for best results use leftover tagliatelle or linguine).
2. Gently heat the olive oil in a 30 cm (12 inch) saucepan.
3. Stir in the pasta in the saucepan for 5 minutes mixing frequently.
4. Add the tomato sauce. It should be just enough to give a bit of coloring but it is important that the mixture remains as dry as possible.
5. In a bowl break and beat the eggs, and add salt and pepper.
6. Pour the mixture over the pasta, reduce the heat, mix gently for 1 minute and then let it settle for 3 minutes.
7. Place a plate on the pan, turnover the pan keeping the plate under it, remove the pan and gently slide the uncooked side of the frittata back into the pan. Cook for another 5 minutes until the eggs are cooked throughout.
8. Remove from the heat and keep covered for 10 minutes.
9. Cut into wedges and serve warm or cold.

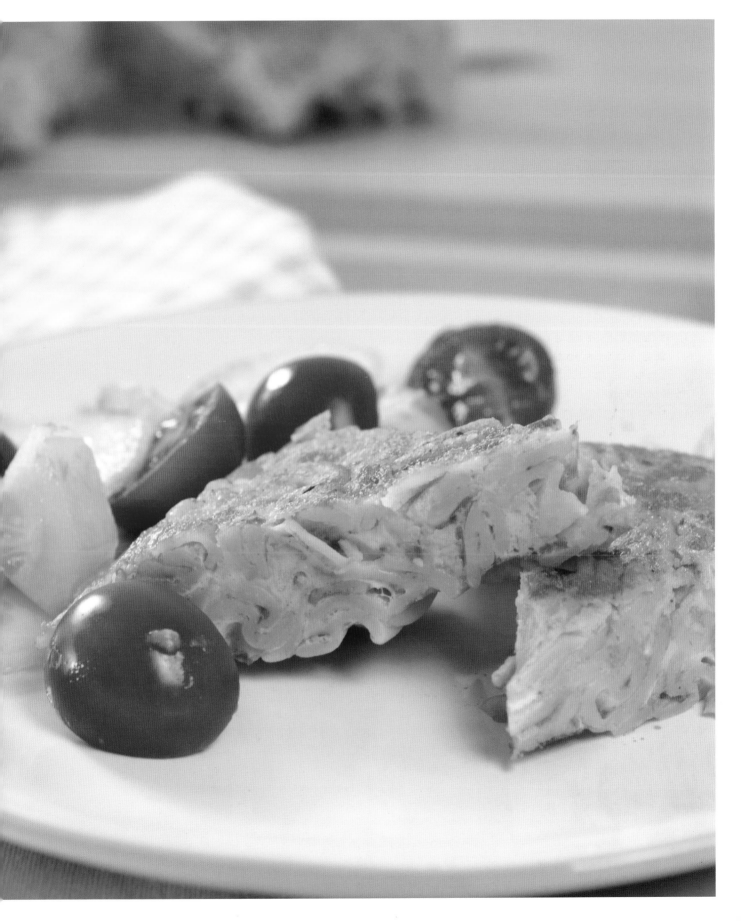

ASPARAGUS AND SWEET PEA RISOTTO

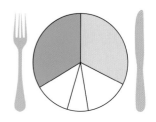

This comforting and creamy green risotto is simple to make and is packed with masses of nutrients and flavors. The sweetness of the peas blends beautifully with the nutty flavor of fresh asparagus, while starchy risotto rice nicely brings all the ingredients and flavors together. Asparagus is rich in energizing B vitamins and chromium that enhances the ability of insulin to transport glucose from the bloodstream into cells while sweet peas are a good source of protein and fiber. Although very creamy, there is no cream, cheese or butter in this dish – creaminess is purely down to constant stirring while cooking. Rice, when stirred, slowly releases the starches which, when combined with the broth, create a thick and cream-like sauce.

■ Fruit & Vegetables
☐ Carbohydrates
☐ Milk, Dairy or Alternatives
☐ High in Sugar and/or Fat
☐ Proteins

2 tbsp olive oil
3 shallots, finely chopped
1 garlic clove, finely chopped
1 handful of fresh basil, finely chopped
150 g (5 oz) fresh asparagus tips, chopped
250 g (9 oz) risotto rice
1 liter (1 ¾ pint) vegetable stock
1tbsp fresh lemon juice
Salt and freshly ground black pepper

Serves: 4
Preparation Time: 10 min
Cooking Time: 30 min

1. Heat the oil in a casserole type saucepan on a medium heat, add shallots and gently fry for 2 minutes or until soft and slightly browned.
2. Add finely chopped garlic and basil and fry on a low heat for a further 3 minutes. Add chopped asparagus tips and cook for a further 5 minutes, stirring occasionally.
3. Add risotto rice and cook for a further 3 minutes or until the grain becomes clear half way.
4. Reduce the heat and slowly start adding the vegetable stock, one ladle-full at a time, stirring constantly, until the stock is absorbed.
5. Repeat, stirring constantly, until you obtain a very creamy and oozy texture. Be careful not to overcook the rice and ensure that the overall texture is slightly looser than you think you want it.
6. Add lemon juice, gently stir and serve warm with a drizzle of olive oil.

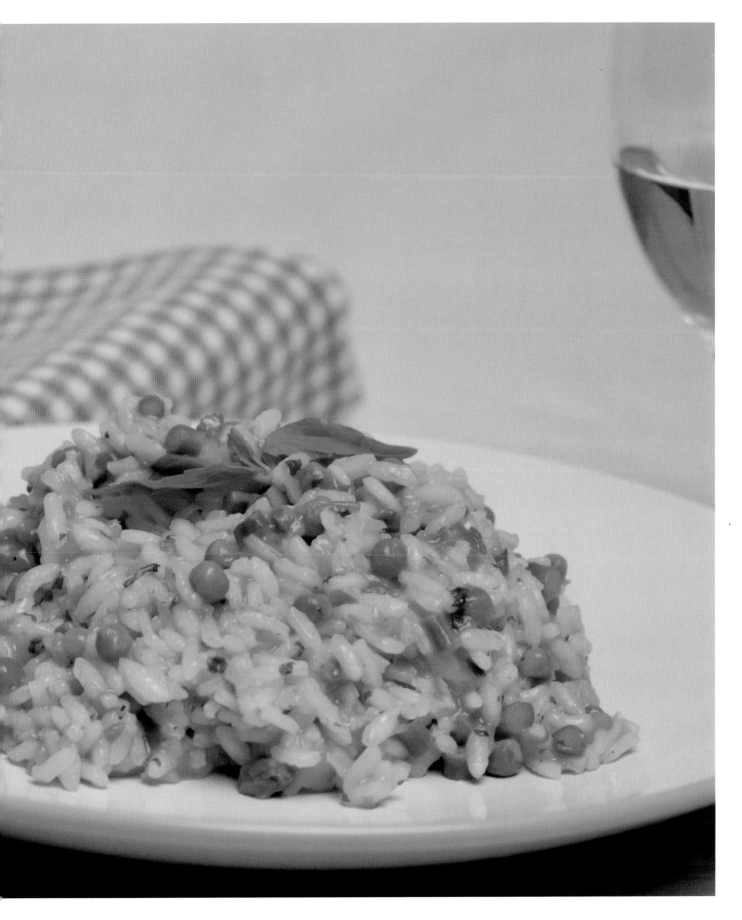

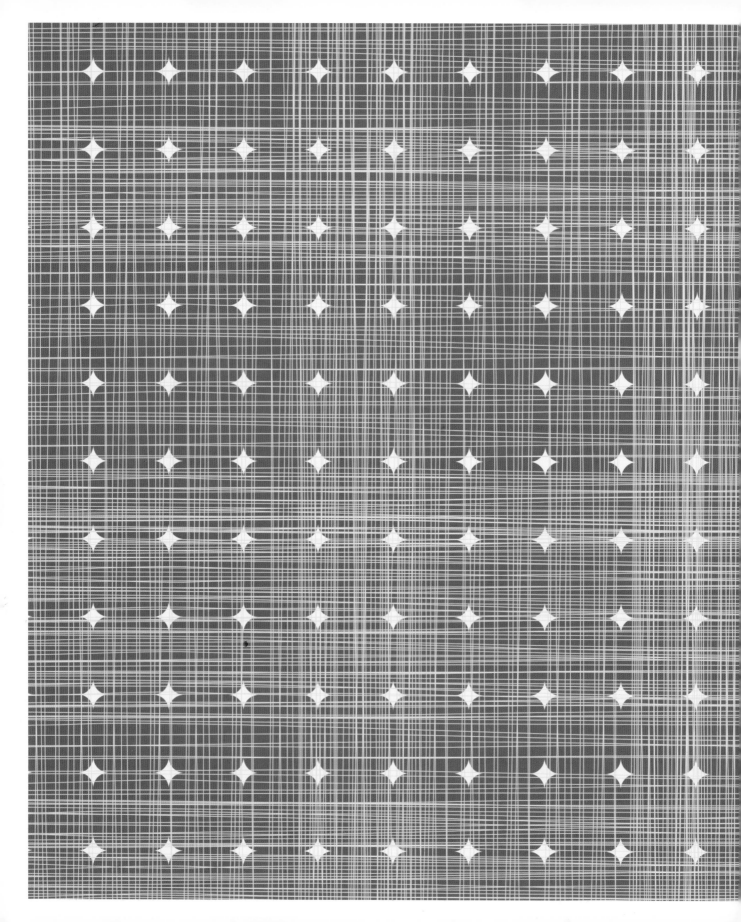

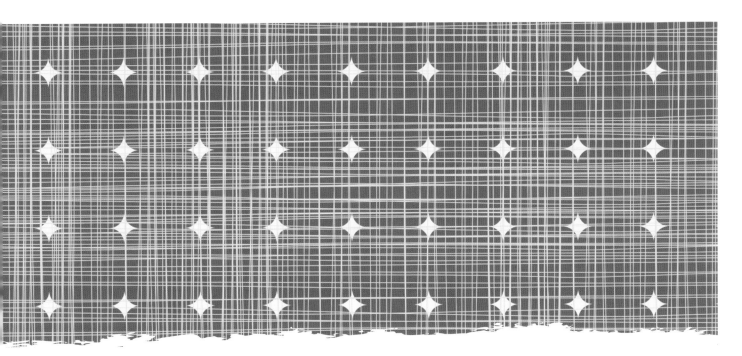

DESSERTS

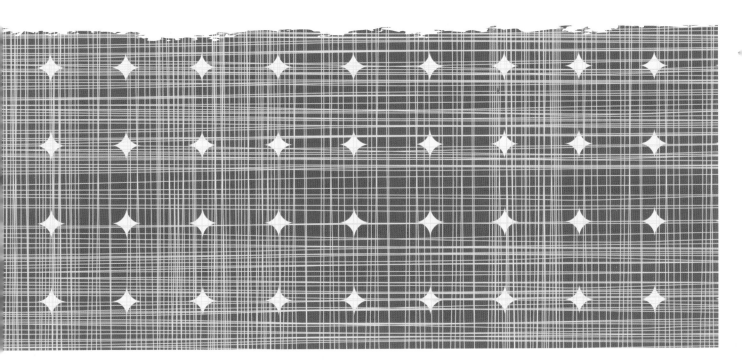

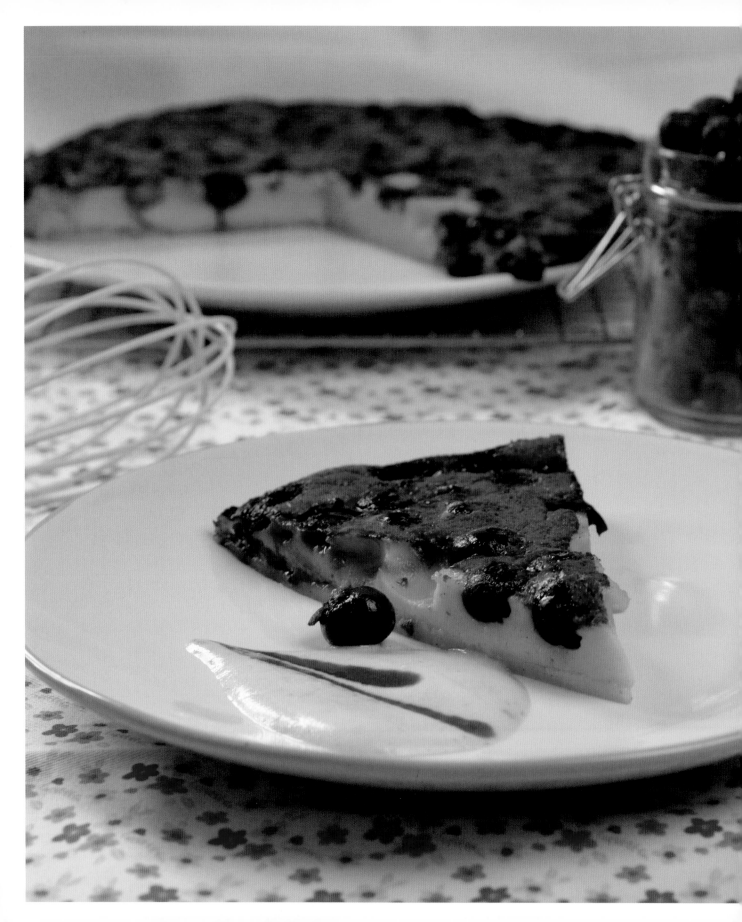

BLUEBERRY CLAFOUTIS

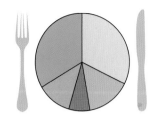

This is a sweetly satisfying, fruity dessert that is equally popular with both, children and adults. Although it contains all the recommended food groups, it's still high in sugars and should be eaten in moderation. You may want to use xylitol instead of sugar as, with a low glycemic index, xylitol has minimal impact on blood glucose levels and may also help to maintain healthy teeth. This just sounds too good to be overlooked!

- ▣ Fruit & Vegetables
- ☐ Carbohydrates
- ▣ Milk, Dairy or Alternatives
- ▣ High in Sugar and/or Fat
- ▣ Proteins

1 tsp coconut oil
75 g (2.5 oz) GF flour
Pinch of salt
90 g (3 oz) raw cane sugar or xylitol
3 eggs
300 ml (10 fl oz) coconut milk
100 ml (3.5 oz) coconut cream
300 g (10 oz) blueberries
1 vanilla pod

Serves 6
Preparation Time: 10 min
Cooking Time: 35 min

1. Preheat the oven to 190°C (375°F).
2. Lightly grease a 25 cm (10 inch) round baking dish with coconut oil.
3. Mix the flour, salt and sugar together. Add the eggs at the center of the mixture, mix well. Combine the coconut milk and coconut cream and slowly beat in the mixture to form a smooth batter.
4. Spread the blueberries on a greased dish, then pour over the batter. Bake for 35 minutes until golden brown.
5. Serve warm or cool.

COCONUT SWIRL

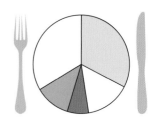

☐ Fruit & Vegetables
☐ Carbohydrates
☐ Milk, Dairy or Alternatives
■ High in Sugar and/or Fat
■ Proteins

My kids can't get enough of these deliciously light and cute looking little swirls. They just magically disappear before my eyes soon after I make them. Needless to say that some of them I very often find cocooned on the back of their toy cars or inside the bear's woolly coat. I still need to keep reminding them that although, these swirls are incredibly tasty, some of their toy friends might not like them as much as they do. These biscuits require minimal ingredients and are really easy and quick to make. The naturally sweet and rich flavor of the coconut blends beautifully with the delightful fragrance of the vanilla paste. I wish all desserts were so unfussy to make.

. . . .

4 egg whites
60 g (2 oz) xylitol or unrefined
*   brown sugar*
140 g (5 oz) desiccated coconut
1 tbsp corn flour
½ tsp vanilla paste

Makes: 20 cookies
Preparation Time: 10 min
Cooking Time: 15 min

1. Preheat oven to 190°C (375°F) and line a baking tray with non-stick parchment paper.
2. In a large mixing bowl, beat the eggs whites and xylitol (or brown sugar) using an electric hand mixer until stiff.
3. Add the coconut, corn flour and vanilla paste and mix gently with a wooden spoon.
4. Put the mixture into a piping bag with a large nozzle and gently squeeze to form a small swirl. Repeat until you use all the mixture. This recipe makes around 20 coconut swirls.
5. Bake for 15 minutes until honey brown.
6. Remove from the oven and leave to cool on the tray for about 5 minutes and then transfer to a rack to cool completely.

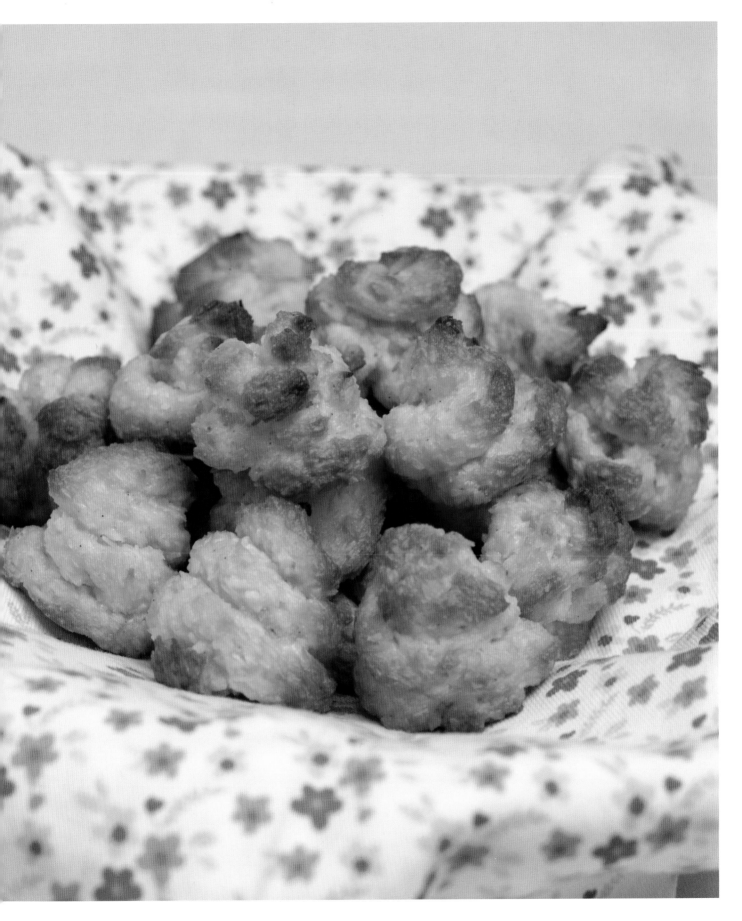

COCONUT PANNA COTTA WITH RASPBERRY AND GOJI BERRY-COULIS

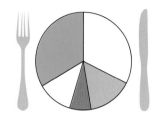

☐ Fruit & Vegetables
☐ Carbohydrates
☐ Milk, Dairy or Alternatives
☐ High in Sugar and/or Fat
☐ Proteins

Wow, what a refreshing little twist! No cow's milk or double cream but yet another one of the most popular Italian classics brought to life. Everyone I know adores this delicate, wobbly, sweetly satisfying, yet incredibly nutritious dessert. The delicious combination of coconut, vanilla and raspberries is just heavenly. This dessert should never be refused.

200 ml (7 fl oz) coconut milk
1 vanilla pod
250 ml (9 fl oz) coconut cream
4 tbsp raw cane sugar or xylitol
3 GF gelatine leaves
30 ml (2 fl oz) raspberry and goji berry coulis (see page 50)

Serves: 4
Preparation Time: 30 min
Cooking Time: N/A

1. For the panna cotta: soak the gelatine leaves in a little cold water for 10 minutes.
2. Place the coconut milk and the vanilla pod into a pan and bring to a simmer. Then remove the pan from the heat and let it rest for a few minutes. Remove the vanilla pod and discard.
3. In a separate pan, mix together the coconut cream and raw cane sugar or xylitol.
4. Squeeze the water out of the gelatine leaves, and then add to coconut cream and sugar or xylitol mixture. Stir well until the gelatine has dissolved.
5. Pour the warm vanilla flavored milk over cream, sugar or xylitol and gelatine mixture, stir well and simmer it on a low heat for 3 minutes.
6. Divide the mixture among 4 pots and leave to cool. Cover the pots with plastic wrap and refrigerate overnight (4 hours minimum).
7. Serve with or without the sauce (see page 50 for raspberry and goji berry coulis recipe).
8. To serve, turn each panna cotta out onto a serving plate, pour over the sauce and garnish with fresh mint and raspberries.

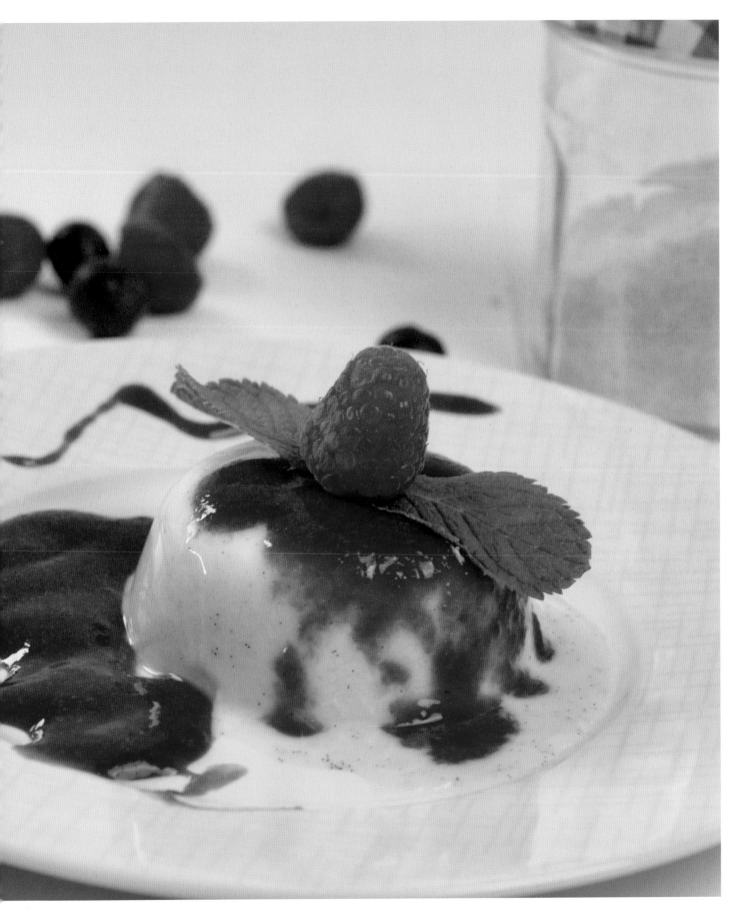

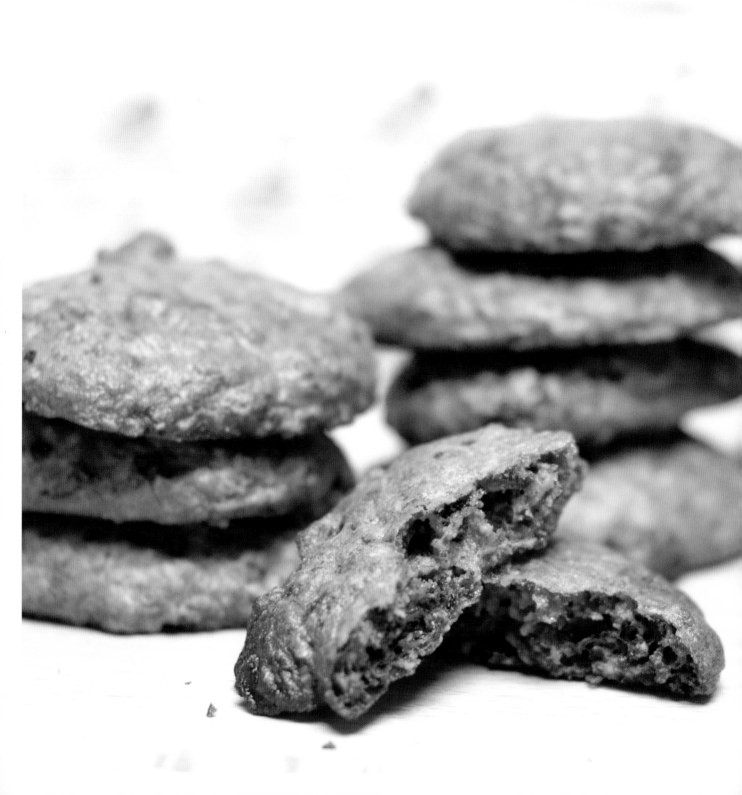

MIDNIGHT COOKIES

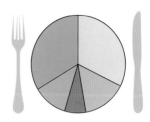

These mysteriously delicious and dark Midnight Cookies are bursting with essential vitamins, fats and minerals. Dates are an excellent energy booster and also provide sweetness and plenty of fiber, iron, and B vitamins while chocolate is a good source of antioxidants, calcium, potassium and A vitamins. On the other hand, the wholemeal rice flour provides plenty of slow-releasing carbohydrates. With no doubt, these are the most flavorsome gluten, dairy, soya and nuts free cookies that I have ever tasted. And not only me, my children can't get enough of them either while my friends don't even realize that they are completely gluten and dairy free.

☐ Fruit & Vegetables
☐ Carbohydrates
☐ Milk, Dairy or Alternatives
☐ High in Sugar and/or Fat
☐ Proteins

60 g (2 oz) coconut oil
40 g (1.5 oz) light brown
  Muscavado sugar
30 g (1 oz) brown granulated sugar
1 egg
½ tsp vanilla bean paste
100 g (3.5 oz) brown rice flour
½ tsp bicarbonate of soda
Pinch of salt
½ tsp xanthan gum
50 g (1.75 oz) DF, GF, SF chocolate,
  chopped (see page 48)
35 g (1 oz) dry dates, chopped

Makes: 15 cookies
Preparation Time: 15 min
Cooking Time: 10 min

1. Preheat oven to 180°C (350°F).
2. In a large bowl, place the coconut oil (oil should be soft but not liquid) and sugar and mix using a hand-held electric mixer until you obtain a creamy mixture. Add an egg and vanilla bean paste and mix again. Add the rice flour, bicarbonate of soda, salt and xanthan gum, mix well.
3. Add the chopped chocolate and dates to form a compact dough.
4. Line a baking tray with non-stick parchment paper.
5. Place 1 teaspoon of the mixture on the tray and shape it with a fork or hand, placing the cookies at least 4 cm (1½ inch) apart so there is enough space for them to expand during the cooking process.
6. Bake for 10 minutes or until dark brown.
7. Remove from the oven and cool in the tray for about 3 minutes and then transfer on a cake grid to cool down completely.
8. Serve slightly warm or cold or keep stored in an airtight container for up to 2 days – if they last that long!

SWEET CHERRY CAKE

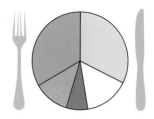

This summery and deliciously moist cake is full of brilliant flavors and nutrients. Cherries are packed with antioxidants and are naturally rich in iron, potassium, vitamin B and vitamin C. They also contain a compound called melatonin, which helps to induce sleep. This dessert has also been sweetened with xylitol, which has a much lower glycaemic index than sugar to help keep blood sugar levels even throughout the day. Eggs are a complete source of protein and are an excellent source of vitamin D, vitamin B12 and selenium.

This incredibly tasty cake is definitely one of the Casa Farina's favorites. It can be enjoyed hot (with a scoop of your favorite ice cream) or cold at any time of the day. This is my favorite midnight snack. Yummy, yum!

- ☐ Fruit & Vegetables
- ☐ Carbohydrates
- ☐ Milk, Dairy or Alternatives
- ☐ High in Sugar and/or Fat
- ☐ Proteins

200 g (7 oz) canned pears in juice, drained (440 g can)
3 eggs
4 tbsp xylitol
½ tsp vanilla pod paste
60 g (2 oz) desiccated coconut
80 g (3 oz) GF flour
1 tsp GF baking powder
¼ tsp xanthan gum
230 g (8 oz) frozen cherries

Serves: 6
Preparation Time: 15 min
Cooking Time: 40 min

1. Preheat oven to 180°C (350°F).
2. Line a loaf baking tray with baking parchment.
3. Place the pears, egg yolks, sugar (xylitol), vanilla bean paste and desiccated coconut into a food processor and process until smooth and creamy.
4. Pour the mixture into a bowl, add the flour, baking powder, xanthan gum and combine all the ingredients.
5. In a separate small bowl, whisk the egg whites with an electric hand mixer until firm and stiff slightly rounded peaks form. Gently fold the egg whites into the pear mixture. Add the frozen cherries and mix gently.
6. Pour the mixture into the baking tray and bake for 40 minutes.
7. Remove from tray and leave to cool on a wire rack.
8. Serve warm or cold.

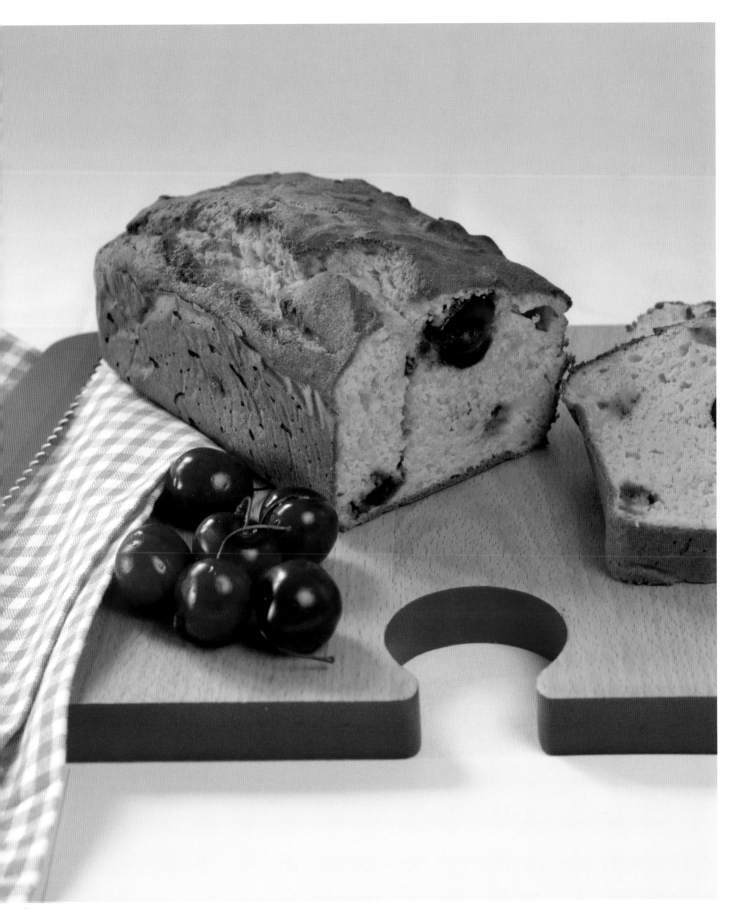

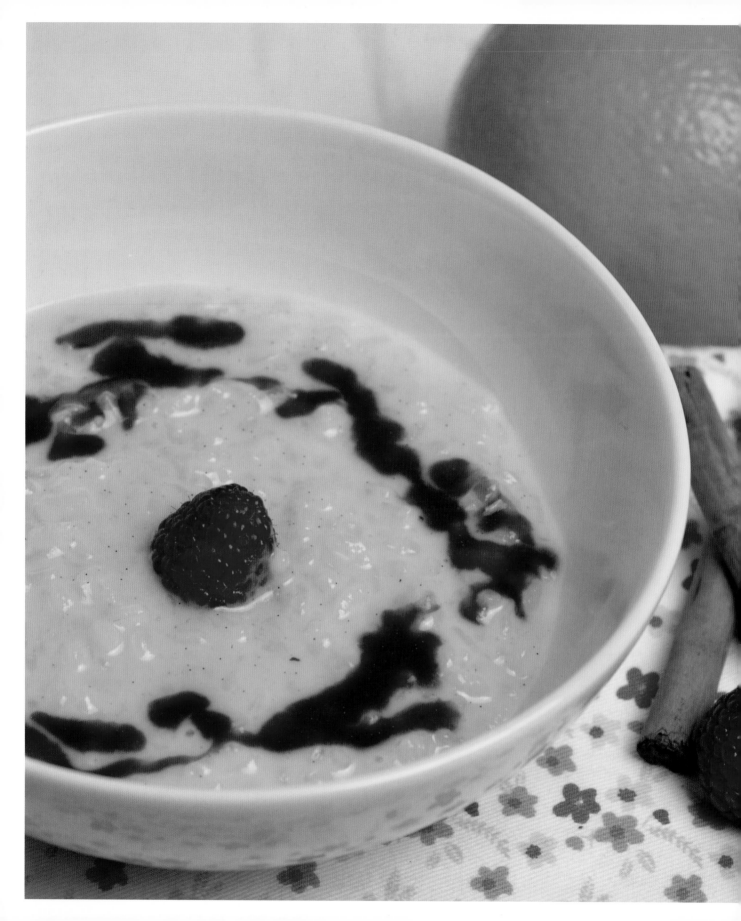

CREAMY RICE PUDDING WITH RASPBERRY AND GOJI BERRY COULIS

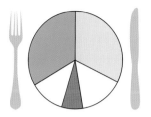

This indulgent and comforting dessert is an all-time favorite. The blend of coconut milk and rice give it a wonderfully rich, smooth and creamy texture. To make it just prefect, add a handful of fresh, sweet and sour raspberries that melt in your mouth. Not only that, the raspberries give it a wonderful summery touch and they are packed with nutrients. Raspberries are rich in antioxidants, soluble fiber, vitamin B and vitamin C.

And don't forget to top it up with sweet and flavorful raspberry and goji berry coulis. Happy indulgence!

- ■ Fruit & Vegetables
- ☐ Carbohydrates
- ☐ Milk, Dairy or Alternatives
- ■ High in Sugar and/or Fat
- ☐ Proteins

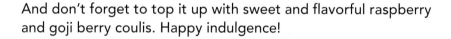

1 liter (1¾ pint) coconut milk
90 g (3 oz) rice for puddings
2 tbsp light brown sugar
1 tsp vanilla pod paste
1 cinnamon stick
Skin of ½ an orange
1 handful of fresh raspberries
Raspberry and goji berry coulis (see page 50)

Serves: 6
Preparation Time: 5 min
Cooking Time: 35 min

1. Place the milk, rice, sugar, vanilla pod paste, cinnamon stick and orange skin into a saucepan, mix well and gently bring to the boil.
2. Reduce heat, cover and simmer gently for 35 minutes or until the rice is cooked, creamy and all the liquid is absorbed.
3. Pour the rice pudding into individual bowls, place a few fresh raspberries on top and swirl the raspberry and goji berry sauce around.
4. Serve immediately.

SWEET MAKI ROLLS

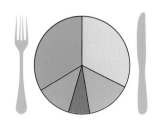

Fruity and chocolaty, these pancake rolls are utterly delicious and packed with masses of nutrients and flavor. You can easily prepare the pancakes in advance and then assemble the makis just before your guests arrive. These maki rolls look very presentable on a plate and are perfect for parties or as a healthy treat too. They are also an easy way to boost your intake of fresh fruits. Blueberries are a wonderful superfood, packed with antioxidants, vitamins C and E, and selenium. Bananas are rich in dietary fiber, B vitamins and potassium while strawberries and raspberries are an excellent source of vitamin C, zinc and antioxidants.

This is as healthy as a dessert can get.

- ☐ Fruit & Vegetables
- ☐ Carbohydrates
- ☐ Milk, Dairy or Alternatives
- ■ High in Sugar and/or Fat
- ☐ Proteins

....

2 pancakes around 26 cm (10 inch) in diameter, (GF, DF and SF see recipe page 49)
30 g (1 oz) chocolate, melted (GF, DF and SF see recipe page 48)
1 fresh banana, cut lengthwise
½ handful fresh blueberries
½ handful fresh raspberries
2 fresh strawberries
30 ml (1 fl oz) fresh whipped cream (see recipe page 51)

Serves: 2
Preparation Time: 10 min
Cooking Time: 15 min (for pancakes)

1. Once the pancakes are ready and cool, assemble your maki following the below instructions.
2. Lay a pancake on a flat surface, spread generously right to the edges with melted chocolate, add cut banana, blueberries, strawberries and raspberries (or a selection of fruits of your choice), roll up tightly, slice into rolls and serve standing to attention, with the cut side down. Add a dollop of fresh whipped cream onto a serving plate and generously glaze with the melted chocolate and scatter a few fresh fruits around to look pretty.
3. Serve immediately.

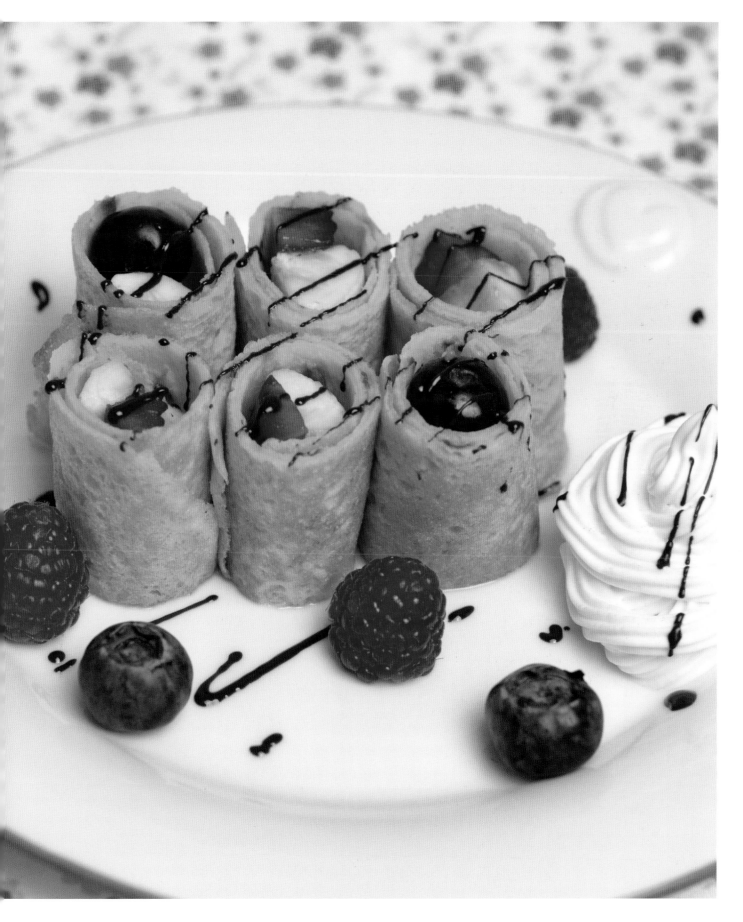

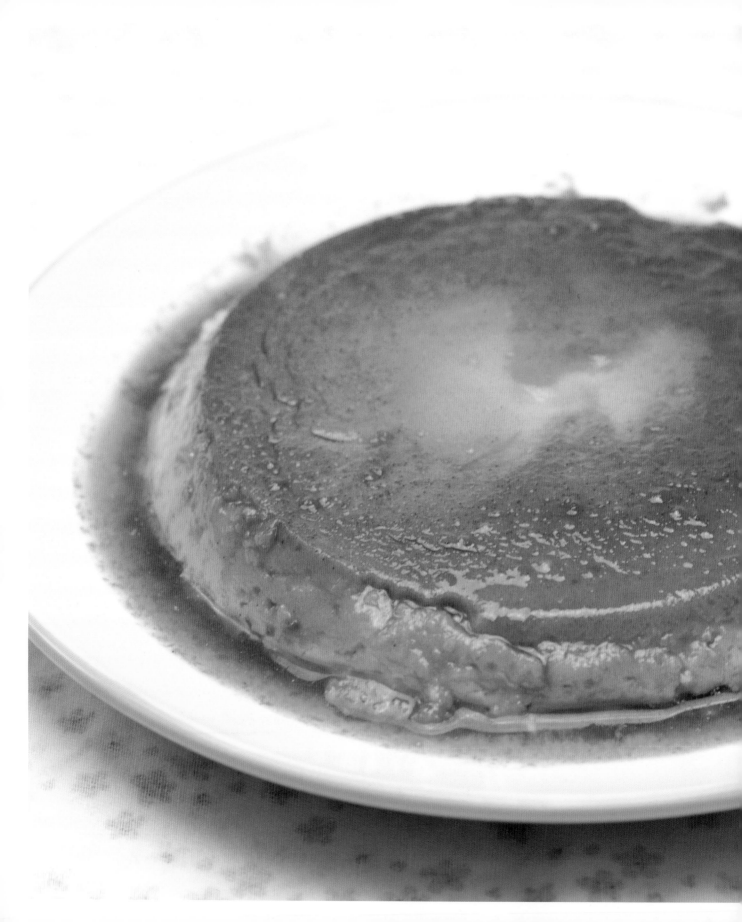

CRÈME CARAMEL

This light and indulgent dessert is a playful twist on the well-known French classic. Simply use a light coconut milk instead of a double cream to create that delightful and wonderfully smooth treat. There is plenty of goodness in this dessert too; eggs are a complete source of protein. Coconut milk is rich in medium-chain saturated fatty acids, antioxidants and immune system boosting A and C vitamins. This wobbly, melt-in-the-mouth dessert will prove irresistibly good to the whole family.

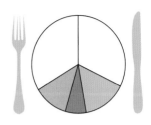

☐ Fruit & Vegetables
☐ Carbohydrates
☐ Milk, Dairy or Alternatives
■ High in Sugar and/or Fat
☐ Proteins

80 g (2.75 oz) light brown unrefined sugar
1 tbsp water
1 tsp vanilla bean paste
500 ml (17 fl oz) light coconut milk
3 eggs
boiling water (used only for hot water bath – quantity depends on the size of the baking tray)

Serves: 6
Preparation Time: 10 min
Cooking Time: 35 min

1. Preheat oven to 160°C (320°F).
2. Warm a baking pot or the ramekins in the oven so that they are warm when the caramel is poured in.
3. Place 30 g (0.75 oz) of light brown unrefined sugar and one tablespoon of water in a stainless saucepan and bring to the boil on a low heat. Do not stir the caramel, wait until the sugar becomes light brown in color and melts completely and then remove immediately from the heat to ensure the caramel does not burn.
4. Quickly pour the caramel into the warmed baking pot or the ramekins ensuring that the bottom of the mould and its sides are fully coated with caramel.
5. In a separate saucepan, place the milk and vanilla bean paste and bring to the boil. Remove from heat and put aside.
6. In a small bowl, whisk the eggs well with the remaining 50 g (2 oz) of sugar. Gently pour the hot milk and vanilla bean paste mixture into the egg and sugar mixture, stirring constantly.
7. Pour the mixture into the caramel coated baking moulds (baking pot or ramekins) and place in a baking tray. Carefully pour the boiling water into the baking tray until ⅔ of the way up the sides of the baking pot or the ramekins. Cover the baking tray with aluminum foil and bake in the hot water bath (bain-marie) for 35 minutes or until the custard is fully set.
8. Remove from the oven and carefully remove the baking pot or ramekins from the water bath. Let stand at room temperature for 4–5 minutes and then refrigerate until well chilled.
9. To serve, run a sharp knife around the baking pot, invert the crème caramel onto a serving plate and serve immediately.

COCONUT AND CHOCOLATE COOKIES

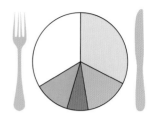

□ Fruit & Vegetables
□ Carbohydrates
▣ Milk, Dairy or Alternatives
■ High in Sugar and/or Fat
▣ Proteins

Unlike many other traditional crispy and hard cookies, these delicious cookies are soft, slightly crumbly and incredibly tasty. They are packed with antioxidants and are an excellent energy booster. They form a good combination when served with a lovely cup of tea/coffee on those long and chatty Sunday afternoons and are also a perfect choice for those with fewer teeth, young or old. My kids love them with a glass of milk and due to its chocolaty color (thanks to a raw cocoa powder), they always eat them so proudly thinking they are eating their favorite chocolate cookies.

150 g (5 oz) GF flour
1 tbsp baking powder
80 g (3 oz) desiccated coconut
50 g (1.75 oz) caster sugar
100 g (3.5 oz) xylitol or unrefined
   brown sugar
½ tsp salt
2 eggs
1 tsp vanilla bean paste
50 g (1.75 oz) coconut oil
2 tbsp coconut milk
1 tbsp raw cacao powder

Makes: 12 cookies
Preparation Time: 10 min
Cooking Time: 10 min

1. Preheat oven to 180°C (350°F) and lightly grease a baking tray. In a large bowl, stir together the flour, baking powder, desiccated coconut, coconut milk, cacao powder, caster sugar, xylitol or unrefined brown sugar and salt. Make a well in the center and add eggs, vanilla paste and coconut oil and mix thoroughly with a wooden spoon.
2. Divide dough into small 24 pieces or bigger 12 pieces, flatten slightly with a fork and place about 4 cm apart on a baking tray.
3. Bake for 10 minutes or until chocolaty brown – these cookies are not crisp and crunchy but nicely soft and slightly crumbly.
4. Cool slightly on the baking tray before transferring to a wire rack to cool completely.

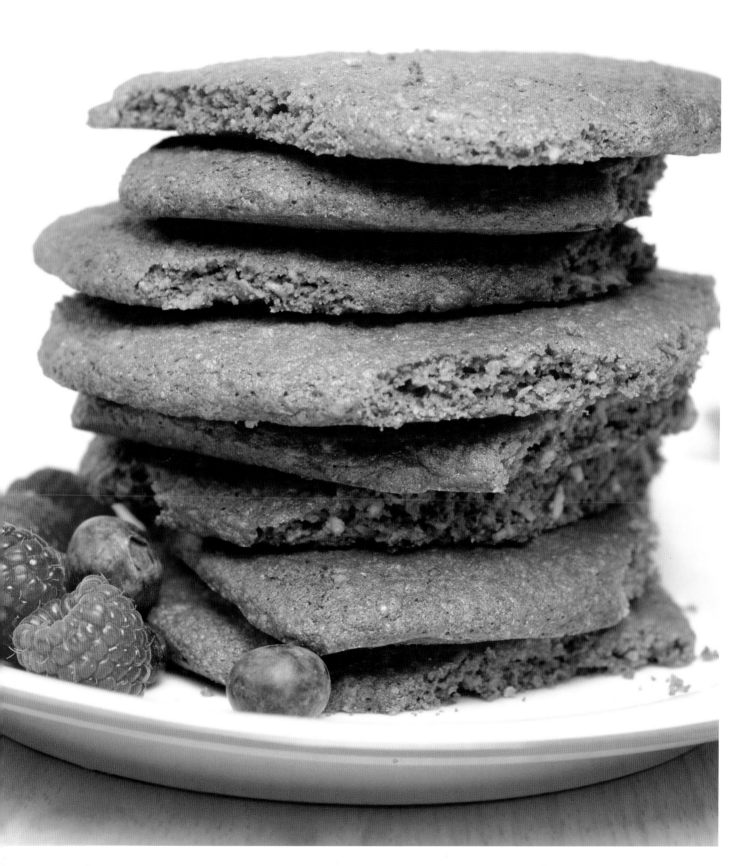

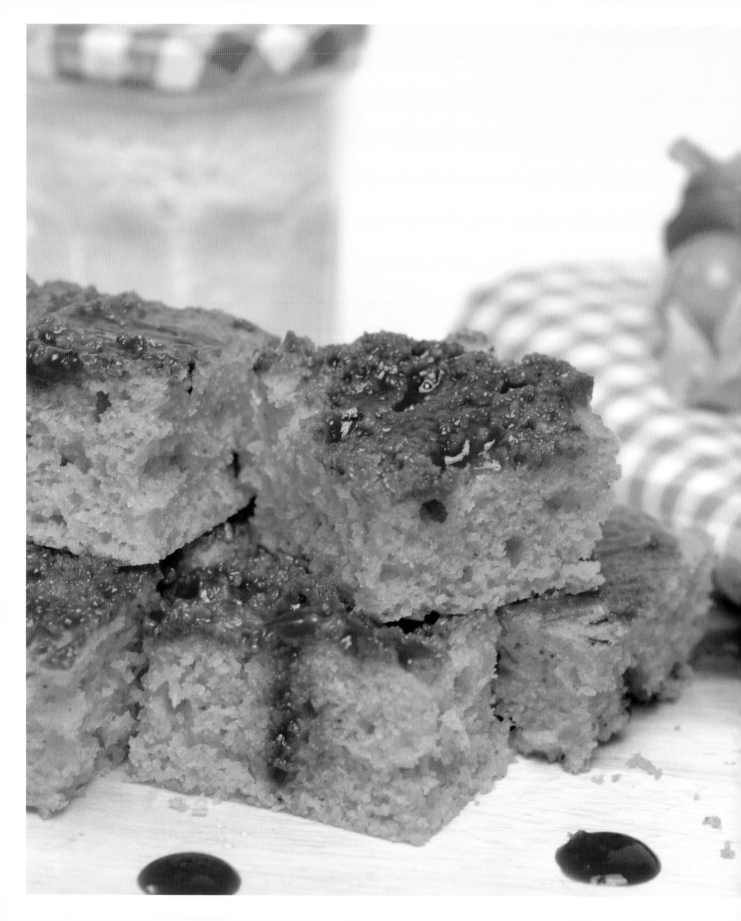

STEAMED COCONUT CAKE WITH RASPBERRY GLAZE

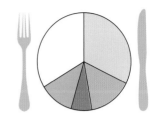

☐ Fruit & Vegetables
☐ Carbohydrates
▣ Milk, Dairy or Alternatives
■ High in Sugar and/or Fat
▣ Proteins

A wonderfully magical combination of coconut and raspberries makes this cake one of my favorite weekend treats. It's steamed; it's light and is truly delicious, perfect accompanier to your cup of tea. You may want to serve it with fresh strawberries and/or raspberries or if you want to bring this indulgence to another level, add a scoop of ice cream (always dairy, soya, nuts and gluten free) Enjoy while your favorite TV series is running in the background. Ah, life is just so beautiful!

. . . .

2 eggs
60 g (2 oz) xylitol or unrefined brown sugar
40 g (1.5 oz) coconut oil
50 ml (1.75 fl oz) coconut milk
115 g (4 oz) GF self-rising (self-raising) flour
½ tsp baking powder
3 tbsp dry unsweetened coconut
4 tbsp raspberry glaze
1 handful of toasted coconut flakes
A pinch of salt

Serves: 4
Preparation Time: 10 min
Cooking Time: 30 min

1. Take a 20 cm (8 inch) steamer basket and line it with the baking parchment.
2. Crack the eggs and separate egg whites from yolks.
3. In a medium size bowl, whisk the egg whites with salt until stiff.
4. Gradually whisk in the sugar, 1 tablespoon at a time, whisking hard after each addition until the mixture forms stiff peaks.
5. Whisk in the yolks and quickly stir in the coconut oil and coconut milk.
6. Sift the self-rising flour and baking powder over the mixture and fold in lightly and evenly with a large metal spoon. Add the dry unsweetened coconut and mix thoroughly.
7. Spoon the mixture into the lined steamer basket and cover it with the spare paper over the top.
8. Place the basket over boiling water, then cover and steam for 30 minutes.
9. Transfer the cake to a plate, remove the paper and let cool slightly. Brush it over with a raspberry glaze and sparingly sprinkle with the coconut flakes. Serve warm or cold.

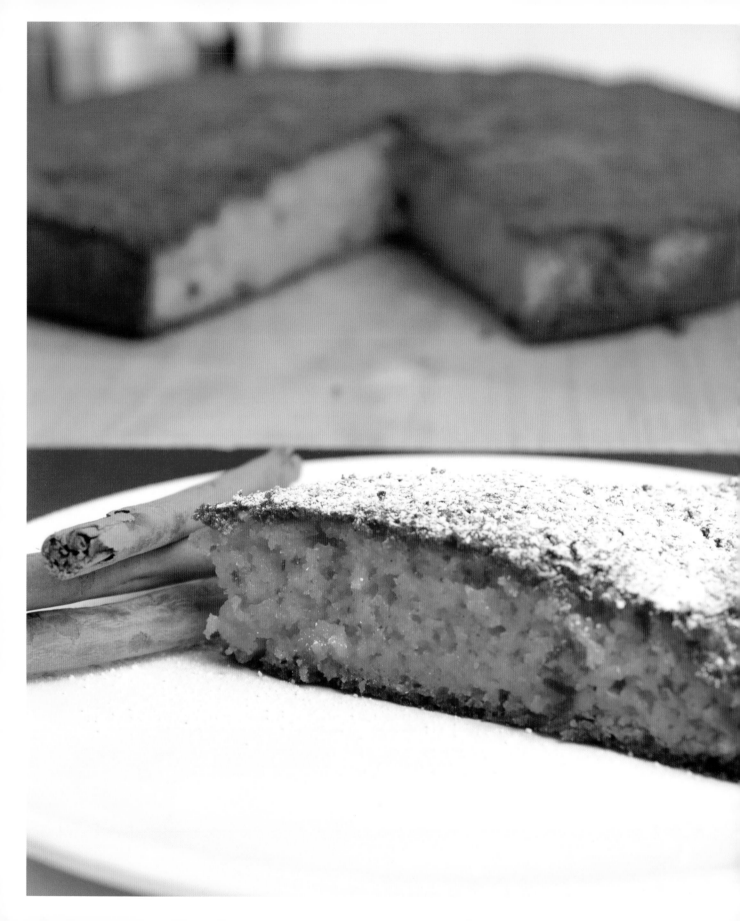

MODERN APPLE AND CARROT CAKE

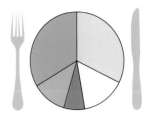

Light, moist and super tasty – this is a healthy twist on an all-time favorite. It's far lower in sugar than traditional apple and carrot cake and it also excludes an old fashioned and highly calorific cream cheese frosting. This is a steady energy booster, good for anytime and a guaranteed hit with the whole family.

☐ Fruit & Vegetables
☐ Carbohydrates
☐ Milk, Dairy or Alternatives
☐ High in Sugar and/or Fat
☐ Proteins

3 eggs
90 g (3 oz) coconut oil
110 g (4 oz) xylitol or raw cane sugar
½ tsp grated nutmeg
150 g (5 oz) grated carrots
100 g (3.5 oz) grated apple
1 tbsp vanilla bean paste
1 tbsp ground cinnamon
1 orange grated zest
100g (3.5 oz) GF self-rising (self-raising) flower
75 g (2.75 oz) corn flour
50 g (1.75 oz) flaked coconut
Icing sugar for dusting (optional)

Serves: 6
Preparation Time: 20 min
Cooking Time: 45 min

1. Preheat the oven to 180°C (350°F) and lightly grease a 25 cm (10 inch) round baking dish with coconut oil.
2. In a separate medium-size bowl, combine: eggs yolks, coconut oil and sugar (xylitol or raw cane) and mix well.
3. Stir in grated nutmeg, carrots and apples, vanilla bean paste, cinnamon, and orange zest and mix thoroughly.
4. Combine the GF flour, corn flour and flaked coconut and slowly beat in the mixture.
5. Beat the egg white with a food processor in a separate bowl.
6. Add the egg white to the mixture to form a smooth batter.
7. Pour the mixture into the greased dish and bake for 45 minutes.
8. Leave to rest.
9. Powder with icing sugar (optional).
10. Serve cool.

CHOCOLATE MOUSSE WITH BLUEBERRIES

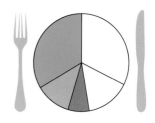

This is an indulgent and rich chocolate dessert made in minutes, without any flour, sugar, eggs, dairy, soya or nuts but with plenty of healthy nutrients and tons of flavor. This really does sound too good to be true, but the richness and smoothness of avocado, the bitterness of raw cocoa powder and the sweetness of date syrup and fresh blueberries blend together to create an irresistibly delicious chocolate dessert loved by all. I like to serve it chilled in a small cute espresso cup, decorated with a piece of fresh fruit.

Raw cacao powder acts as a slight antidepressant by promoting a production of the 'feel good hormones' in the body and is also packed with antioxidants. Avocados are naturally rich in energizing B vitamins and easily digestible monosaturated fats, date syrup is a good source of iron, potassium and magnesium while beautiful blueberries are bursting with vitamins C and E, antioxidants and zinc.

So, I think there is only one more thing I can add: enjoy it guilt-free and, of course, always with a smile!

- ■ Fruit & Vegetables
- ☐ Carbohydrates
- ☐ Milk, Dairy or Alternatives
- ■ High in Sugar and/or Fat
- ■ Proteins

Serves: 4
Preparation Time: 5 min
+ 30 min chilling
Cooking Time: N/A

....

1 large ripe avocado (peeled, de-stoned and cut into chunks)
50 g (1.75 oz) fresh blueberries
4 tbsp date syrup
40 g (1.5 oz) unsweetened raw cocoa powder
½ tsp vanilla bean paste
3 tbsp coconut milk
Pinch of salt

1. Add all the ingredients into a blender and process to make a thick, rich, mousse-like dessert. Place the mousse into a bowl, cover with plastic wrap, place in the fridge and chill for 30 minutes.
2. Serve in a small espresso cup, decorate with fruits or as desired and serve immediately.

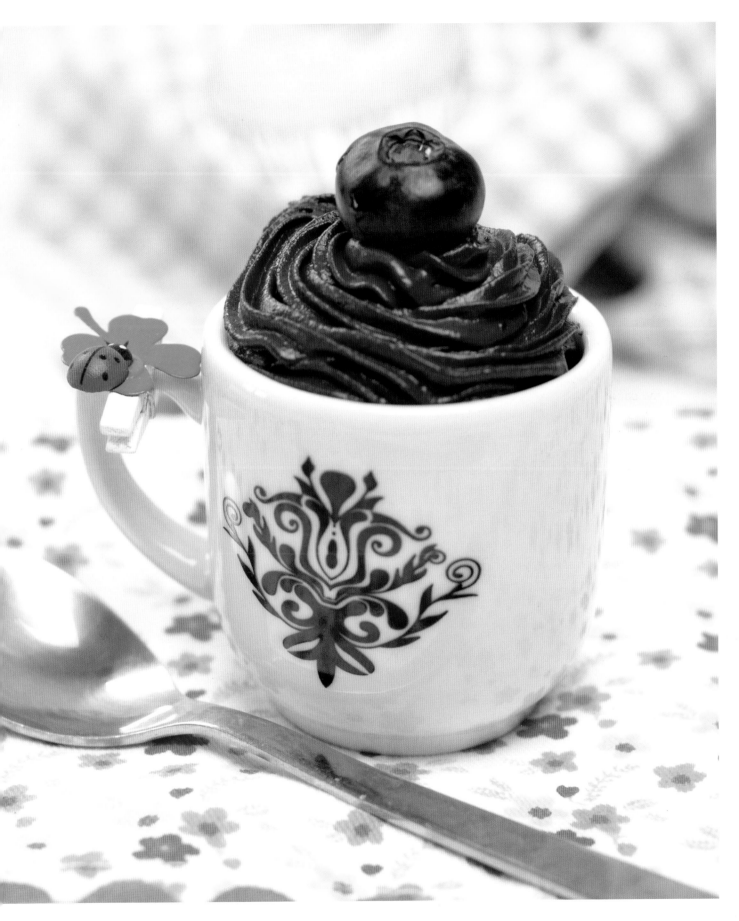

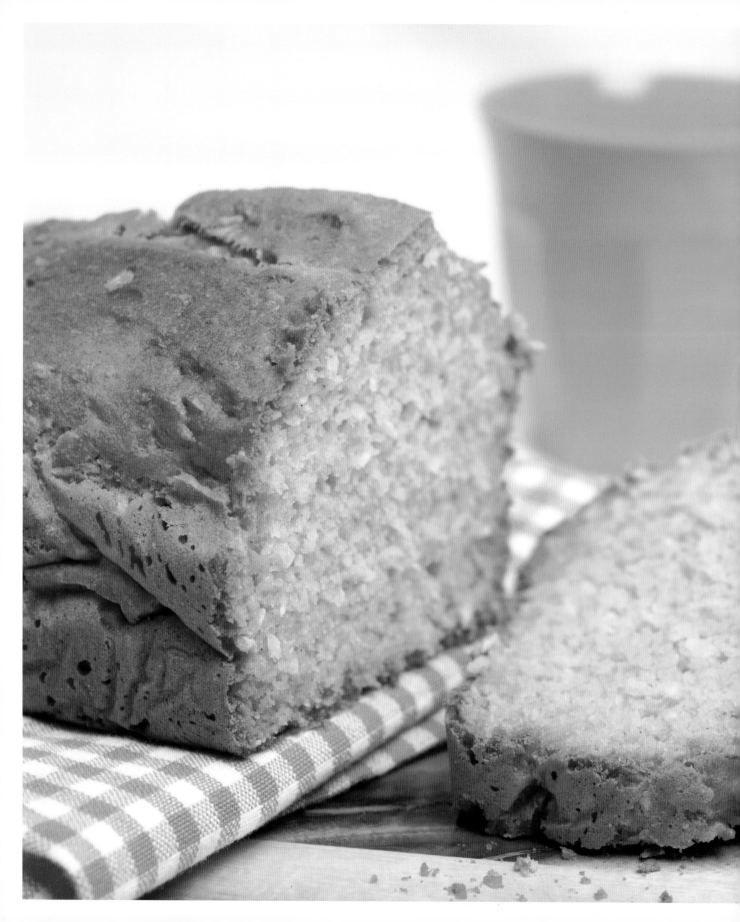

COCONUT LOAF CAKE

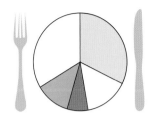

This moist and irresistibly delicious loaf cake is guaranteed to be a hit with the whole family. It's quick and easy to make, delicious and packed with plenty of nutrients and flavors.
Eggs are a complete source of proteins and vitamin D while coconut oil is rich in easily digestible, medium chain fatty acids and dietary fiber.

The flavor and texture of this cake is a perfect complement to your cup of tea. My children love it with a glass of milk in the morning.

☐ Fruit & Vegetables
☐ Carbohydrates
☐ Milk, Dairy or Alternatives
■ High in Sugar and/or Fat
■ Proteins

100 g (3.5 oz) desiccated coconut
200 g (7 oz) GF (if not already enriched with xanthan gum, add ½ teaspoon)
100g (3.5 oz) xylitol or unrefined brown sugar
60 ml (2 oz) coconut oil (unflavored)
3 eggs
200 ml (7 fl oz) light coconut milk
1 tsp vanilla bean paste
1 tsp baking powder

Serves: 8
Preparation Time: 10 min
Cooking Time: 40 min

1. Preheat oven to 180°C (350°F) and underline a loaf baking tray with parchment paper.
2. Put all the ingredients together into a large bowl and mix thoroughly.
3. Spread the mixture into the baking tray and bake for 40 minutes.
4. Once cooked, remove from the oven and place on a resting tray to cool.
5. Serve warm or cold.

CHOCOLATE SOUFFLÉ

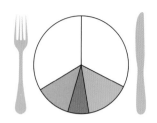

Rich and indulgent, this dessert is always a hit no matter what the occasion. It is packed with proteins, flavonoids, antioxidants and good fats so if eaten in moderation it's not that bad for you. After all, it's still a pudding.

Best served warm with cream and/or fruits.

☐ Fruit & Vegetables
☐ Carbohydrates
◻ Milk, Dairy or Alternatives
◼ High in Sugar and/or Fat
◻ Proteins

---

130 g (4.5 oz) dark chocolate (DF and SF see recipe page 48) melt 100 g (3.5 oz) and divide 30 g (1 oz) into 8 squares
3 eggs
70 g (2.5 oz) xylitol or unrefined brown sugar
20 g (0.75 oz) coconut oil
20 g (0.75 oz) olive oil

Serves: 4
Preparation Time: 10 min
Cooking Time: 10 min

1. Preheat oven to 190°C (375°F).
2. Melt the chocolate over hot water bath (bain marie).
3. Place the eggs, sugar, coconut oil and olive in a bowl and mix well. Pour in melted chocolate and gently mix to combine all the ingredients.
4. Fill up four ramekins halfway. Place two solid chocolate squares on top and cover with the remaining chocolate mixture.
5. Bake for 15 minutes.
6. Once ready, serve immediately. Best served with whipped cream or your favorite ice cream.

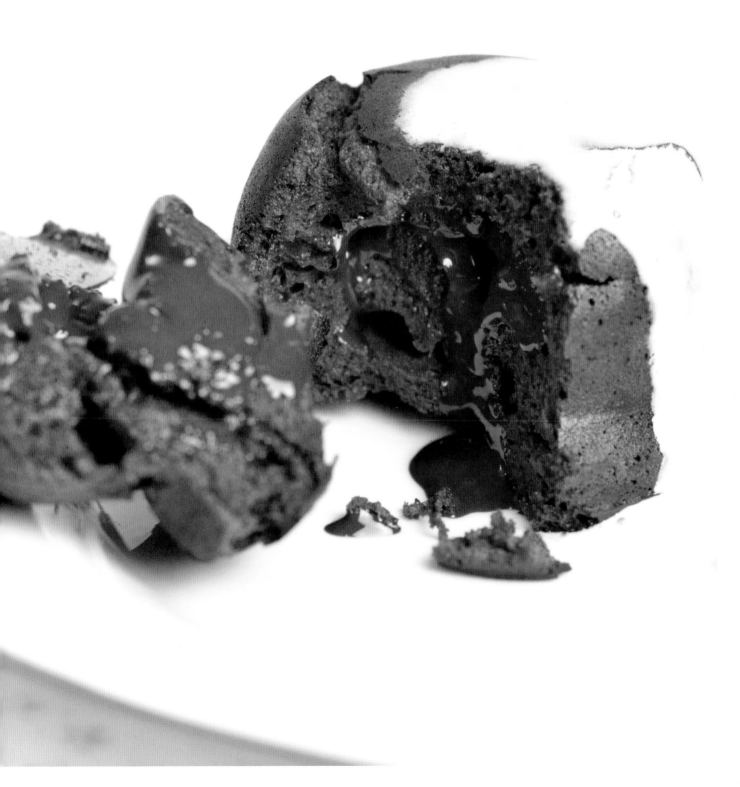

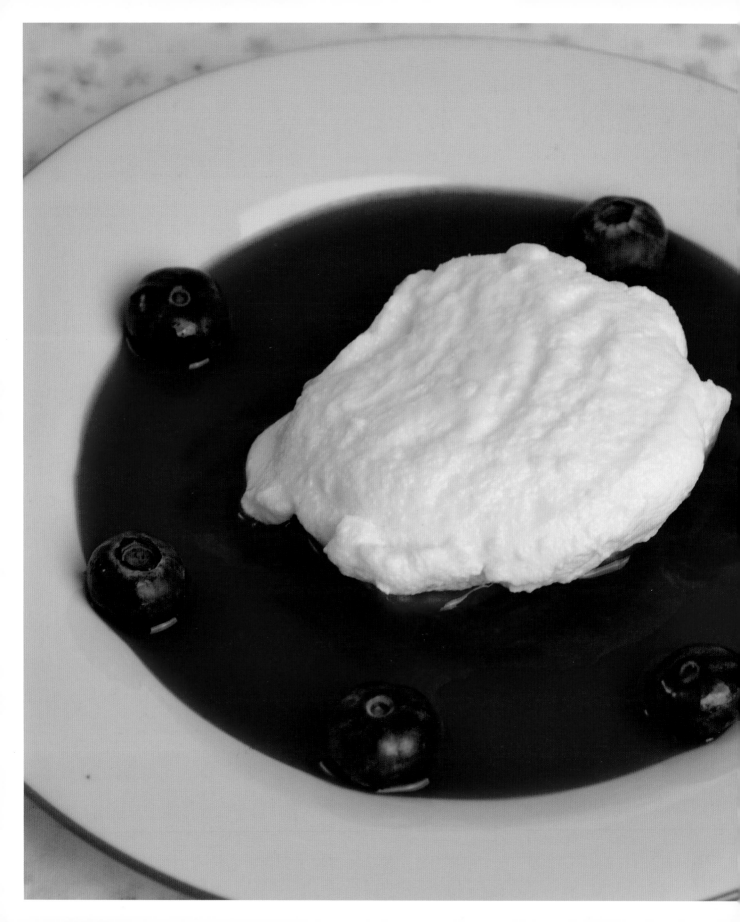

EGG WHITE SNOW BALLS DELIGHT WITH RASPBERRY COULIS

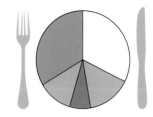

- ▣ Fruit & Vegetables
- ☐ Carbohydrates
- ▣ Milk, Dairy or Alternatives
- ■ High in Sugar and/or Fat
- ▢ Proteins

This comforting dessert is irresistibly delicious and yet so easy to prepare. It is a big hit with my family every time and it also looks very presentable on a plate. My children like to think they are eating snow on the plate.

Egg whites are a good source of protein and unlike egg yolks, are completely free of cholesterol. They also contain small amounts of vitamin B and are generally healthier as the calories and nutrients that you receive from egg whites are of much higher quality than that of whole eggs.

. . . .

4 egg whites
70 g (2.5 oz) xylitol
570 ml (19fl oz) light coconut milk
90 ml (3 fl oz) raspberry coulis – 30 ml (1 fl oz) per portion
30 g (1 oz) blackberries

Serves: 4
Preparation: 10 min
Cooking Time: 5 min

1. Separate the egg whites and keep the egg yolks aside for making another dish such as vanilla custard.
2. In a stainless steel bowl, beat the egg whites until stiff using a hand-held electric mixer or a balloon whisk.
3. Add the sugar and beat again until firm.
4. In a separate casserole type pan, bring the coconut milk to a boil.
5. With two large cooking spoons, form the snowballs, out of the egg white mixture, delicately place them on the hot coconut milk and poach for 2 minutes on each side.
6. Drain the balls well and place on a cake cooler until cold.
7. Pour 30 ml (1 fl oz) of raspberry coulis onto each dessert plate, enough to cover the surface of the plate and place the snowball in the center. Decorate with blueberries or other fruits of your choice.
8. Serve cold.

SCRUMPTIOUS CHOCOLATE SQUARES

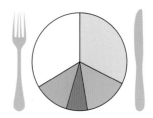

These light and moist chocolate squares are loved by my family, any time of the day, any season and anywhere. It's like they can never have enough of it. And above all, this irresistibly delicious 'no fuss cake' is made in minutes.
Cocoa powder is rich in antioxidants and also helps to increase levels of the 'feel good' hormone serotonin in the brain. This is yet another reason to embark on the chocolate squares adventure trip.

☐ Fruit & Vegetables
☐ Carbohydrates
◩ Milk, Dairy or Alternatives
■ High in Sugar and/or Fat
◩ Proteins

50 ml (1.75 fl oz) light coconut milk
100 g (3.5 oz) xylitol or brown
    unrefined sugar
1 egg
½ tsp vanilla bean paste
80 g (2.75 oz) GF flour
1 tsp baking powder
Pinch of salt
60 g (2 oz) raw cacao powder

Serves: 8 (makes 16 brownies)
Preparation Time: 5 min
Cooking Time: 30 min

1. Preheat oven to 180°C (350°F).
2. In a medium size bowl, mix together coconut milk and unrefined brown sugar or xylitol. Add the egg and vanilla and mix well.
3. Sift together the flour, baking powder and salt and add to the mixture. Blend in raw cacao powder, add coconut milk (light) and mix well.
4. Spread the mixture into a slightly greased baking tray and bake for 30 minutes.
5. Once cooked, remove from the oven and place on a resting tray to cool.
6. Serve warm or cold.

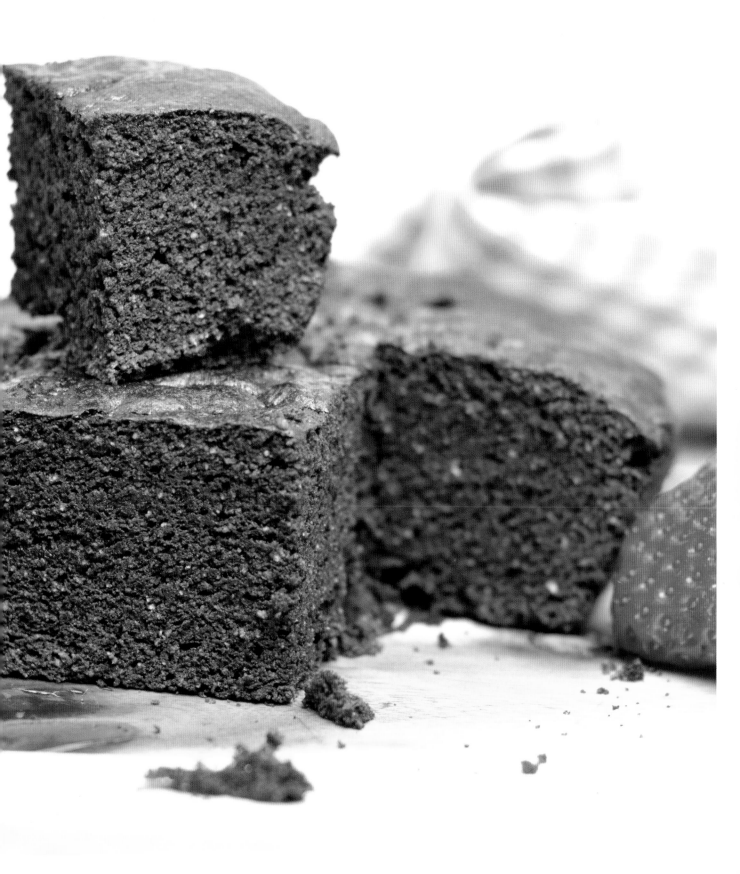

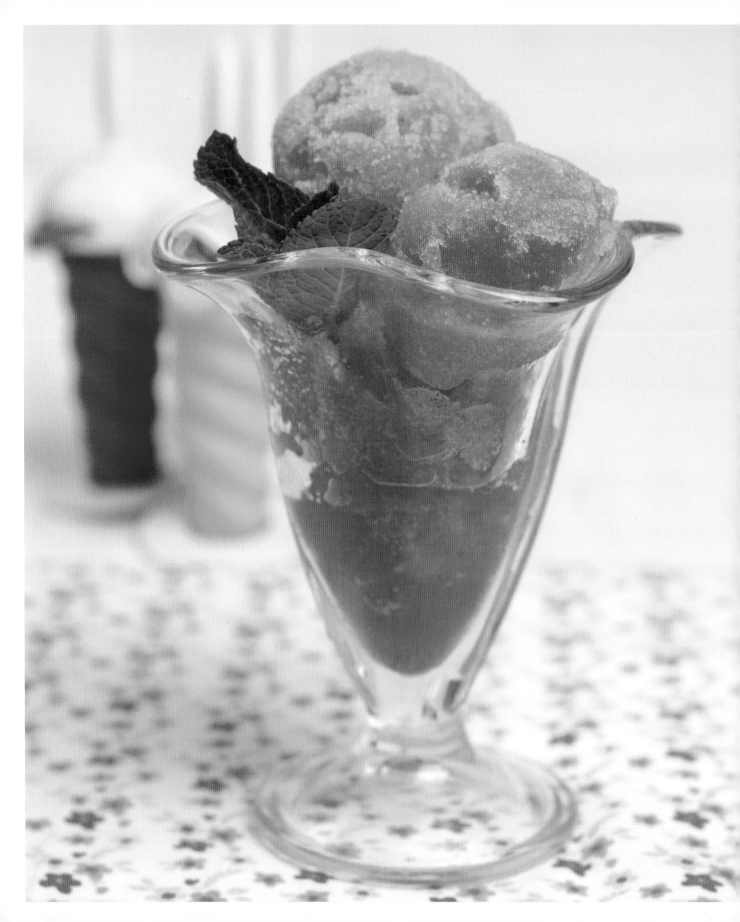

WATERMELON SORBET

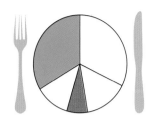

This incredibly refreshing watermelon sorbet is a perfect way to cool down on hot summer days. It also makes a tasty, refreshingly light finish to a meal. Watermelon is naturally packed with masses of nutrients and flavor. It's rich in the antioxidant lycopene that helps fight heart disease and several types of cancer. Watermelon has the highest concentration of lycopene to any other fresh fruit or vegetable. It's also an excellent source of Vitamins A, C and B6 and is rich in potassium, which helps muscle and nerve function. This definitely is one of my favorite fruits of all time. And this sorbet tastes just like eating a slice of fresh watermelon from the farm stand. Just heavenly!

■ Fruit & Vegetables
☐ Carbohydrates
☐ Milk, Dairy or Alternatives
■ High in Sugar and/or Fat
☐ Proteins

200 ml (7 fl oz) water
180 g (6.5 oz) unrefined light brown sugar
1 kg (lb 3 oz) watermelon chunk, seedless
2 tbsp lemon juice

Serves: 6
Preparation Time: 10 min + 40 min resting
Freezing Time: 8 hours

1. In a small saucepan, gently boil the water and sugar, stirring constantly to dissolve the sugar. Once the sugar is dissolved, remove from the heat and put aside to completely cool down.
2. In the meantime, place the seedless watermelon chunks and 2 tablespoons of lemon juice into a blender and gently blend until smooth.
3. Add the sugar mixture into a blender and blend well.
4. Place into an airtight container and freeze for at least 6 hours.
5. Remove from the freezer and leave it at room temperature for 30 minutes to soften, then put into a blender and blend until you obtain a frozen smoothie like texture. Refreeze for at least 2 hours.
6. Before serving, take it out of the freezer, leave it to soften for 10 minutes at room temperature and serve in chilled dishes.

VANILLA CRÈME BRÛLÉE

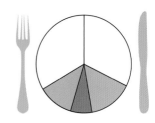

This classic crunchy and custardy delight is always a big hit with the whole family. It's one of those desserts that you think you can never have when you are on a gluten and dairy free diet. But, the reality is very different. Instead of a rich cow milk or double cream, make this irresistibly delicious dessert with thick and sweet flavored coconut cream instead. My guests never notice any difference. Coconut cream is rich in antioxidants, fiber and B vitamins while eggs are a good source of a complete protein. So this is really a 'must have' dessert that is most enjoyable when eaten as a special treat.

☐ Fruit & Vegetables
☐ Carbohydrates
◩ Milk, Dairy or Alternatives
◼ High in Sugar and/or Fat
◩ Proteins

500 ml (17 fl oz) coconut cream
1 tsp vanilla bean paste
5 egg yolks
60 g (2 oz) brown unrefined sugar
6 tsp brown unrefined sugar for sprinkling
water for hot water bath (bain-marie)

Serves: 6
Preparation Time: 15 min
+ 2 hours chilling
Cooking Time: 25 min

1. Preheat the oven to 150°C (300°F).
2. In a saucepan, heat the coconut cream and vanilla paste to just below boiling point. Remove and put aside.
3. In a medium size bowl, cream the egg yolks and sugar, and gradually add the warm cream into the mixture.
4. Pour the mixture into a baking dish or 6 individual ramekins and place into a large baking tray. Carefully pour the water into the baking tray until ⅔ of the way up the sides of the baking dish or the ramekins. Cover the baking tray with aluminum foil and bake in the hot water bath (bain-marie) for 25 minutes.
5. Once ready, carefully take the baking dish or the ramekins out of the bain-marie, let it cool down and then refrigerate for 2 hours.
6. Before serving, sprinkle one teaspoon of brown sugar on top of each ramekin and caramelize using a kitchen torch.
7. Serve warm or cold.

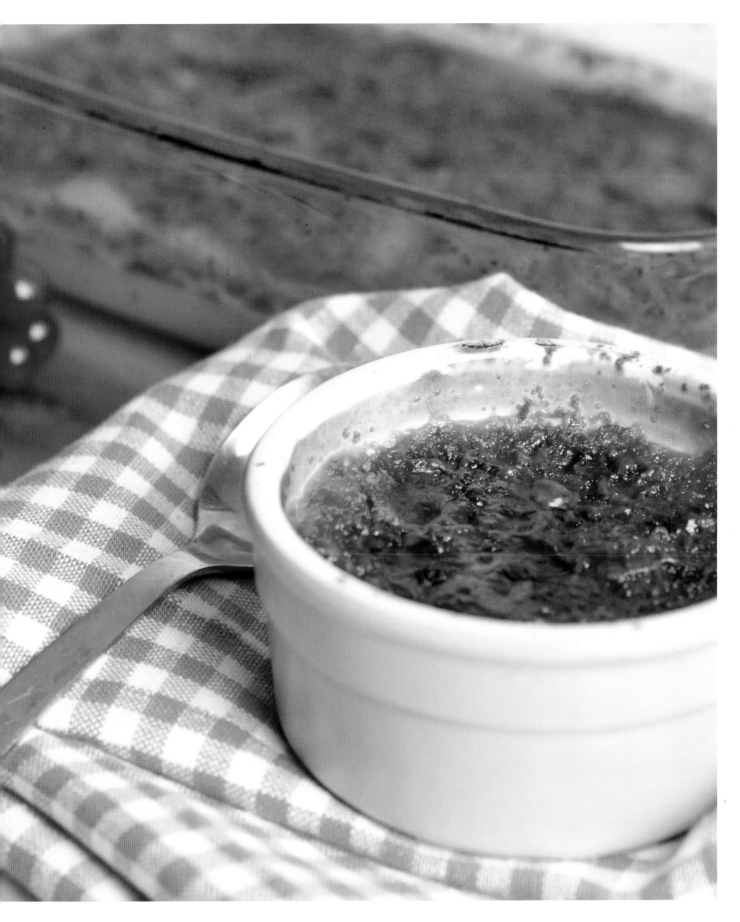

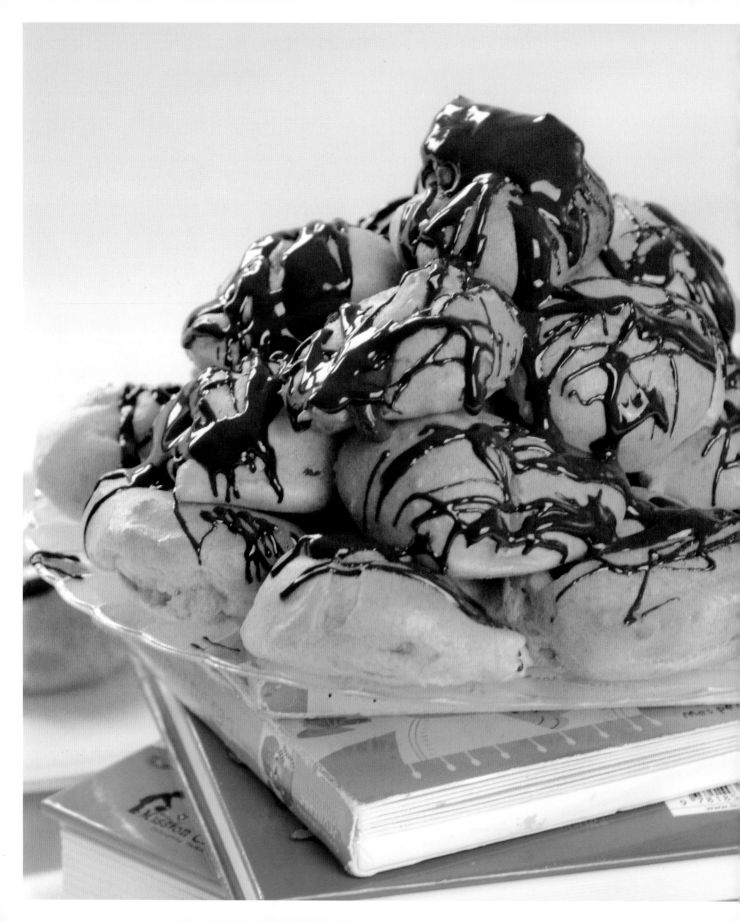

PROFITEROLES WITH CHOCOLATE SAUCE

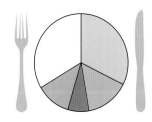

An all-time favorite, this sweetly satisfying dessert is irresistible warm or cold. The filling is wonderfully light, yet creamy and flavorsome. It's no doubt that this dessert is sure to earn cheers of approval from all your family at all times. You may want to add some melted dairy free chocolate into the vanilla custard to create a chocolate filling that is also irresistible.

- ☐ Fruit & Vegetables
- ☐ Carbohydrates
- ☐ Milk, Dairy or Alternatives
- ☐ High in Sugar and/or Fat
- ☐ Proteins

Choux Pastry
250 ml (9 fl oz) water
2 tbsp raw cane sugar or xylitol
70 ml (2.5 fl oz) coconut oil
135 g (4.75 oz) GF flour
A pinch of salt
4 eggs beaten

Vanilla Custard
1 vanilla pod
250 ml (9 fl oz) coconut milk
3 egg yolks
70 g (2.5 oz) raw cane sugar or xylitol
2 tbsp GF flour

Chocolate Sauce
60 g (2 oz) chocolate; GF, DF and SF (see page 48)
1 tbsp coconut milk

Serves: 6 (approx 20 pieces)
Preparation Time: 20 min
Cooking Time: 30 min

1. Preheat the oven to 180°C (350°F).
2. For the Choux Pastry: place the water and sugar and coconut oil into a saucepan and bring to a simmer. Remove the saucepan from the heat and quickly pour in the flour and a pinch of salt and beat the mixture well to form a smooth paste.
3. When the paste stops sticking to the pan, transfer the mixture to a large bowl and leave to cool for 5 minutes. Beat the eggs in, one at a time to form a glossy paste and soft dropping consistency.
4. Cover a baking tray with non-stick paper. Using 2 spoons or a piping bag, align 3 cm (1¼ inch) balls of the mixture on the baking sheet, leaving at least 2 cm (¾ inch) between each ball. Bake for 30 minutes until golden brown. Leave it to rest.
5. For the vanilla custard: slice open the vanilla pod, put into a large saucepan with the coconut milk and bring to boil. Remove from heat.
6. In the meantime, beat the egg yolk and sugar to form a smooth mixture. Add the flour and mix thoroughly. Pour in the milk, mix and transfer the batter back into the pan. Gently bring to the boil, mixing vigorously until the mixture thickens to form the custard. Cover and leave to cool for 15 minutes.
7. Fill in each profiterole with the custard using a piping bag and arrange the filled profiterole on a round plate to form a pyramid.
8. For the Chocolate Sauce: put the chocolate pieces and coconut milk into a small saucepan, gently stir on a low heat until chocolate is almost melted. Remove from the heat, continue mixing until the chocolate is melted.
9. Generously pour the chocolate sauce over the pyramid. Refrigerate for at least 1 hour.

DISCLAIMER

Please remember that any guidance provided in this book is not intended as a substitute for professional medical advice and treatment. The author of this book cannot accept any responsibility for any errors or omissions, inadvertent or not, that may be found in the recipes or text or for any problems that may arise as a result of preparing one of these recipes or following the advice contained in this work.

ACKNOWLEDGEMENTS

My special thank you goes to my wonderful, supportive husband Lorenzo, my best friend, my soulmate, who made this book possible and to my beautiful sons, Leonardo and Nikola, who were always by my side, tirelessly tasting all the brand new gluten, dairy, soya and nut free treats. Thank you for your constant encouragement, support and love throughout this journey. I wholeheartedly dedicate this book to you.

I would also like to thank everyone at New Holland Publishers, especially Holly Willsher, my editor and Diane Ward, my publisher, for their kindness, professionalism and ongoing support with this book.

Thank you to all my family and friends – my mother, Kata, my father, Milan, and my three beautiful sisters (Vesna, Sunčica and Spomenka) for always being there for me. Thank you to my mother in-law, Maria-Grazia, for sharing some inspiring, traditional recipes.

I am also grateful to my university tutor, Dr Bernard Lamb, for his enthusiastic and continuous support and encouragement.

Thank you all for your endless support.

INDEX

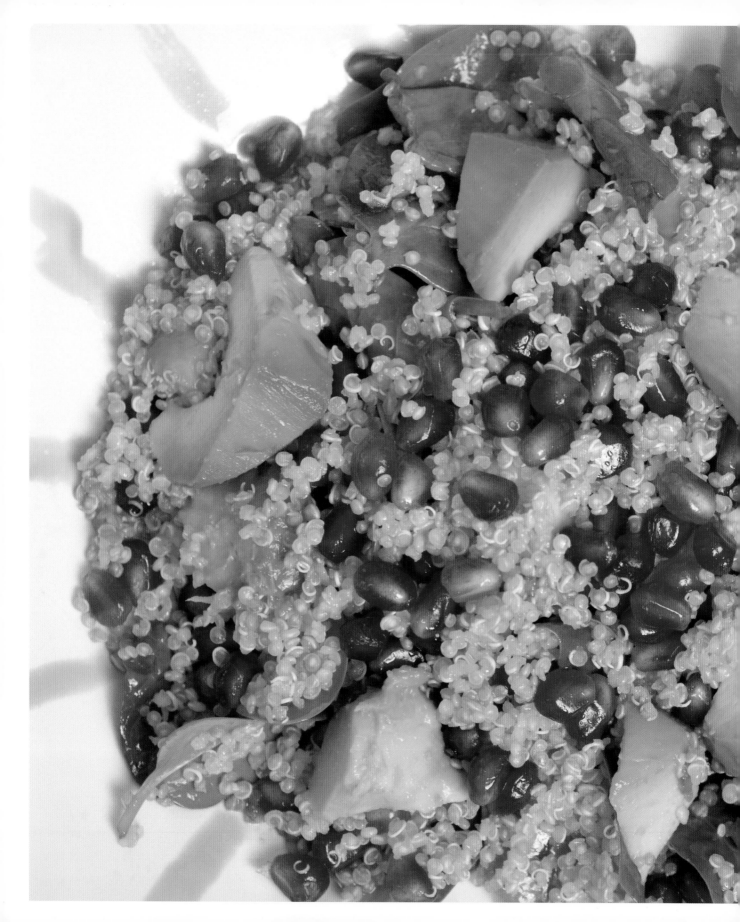

ABOUT THE AUTHOR

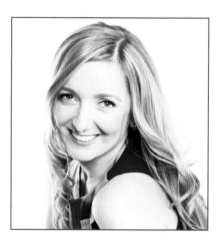

Nada Farina née Matić is a scientist, passionate food enthusiast with an extensive knowledge of nutrition, mother of two young children with food intolerances. She is passionate about nutrition and strongly believes in the beneficial effects of organically grown foods. Nada is currently pursuing an MSc in Human Nutrition in London.

While studying Immunology at Imperial College, she has also gained a scientific knowledge of food hypersensitivities where, in some instances, even a good and healthy food is being rejected by our immune system. Nowadays, food intolerances are on the increase especially amongst young children including her own. When her children were diagnosed with food intolerances to dairy, gluten, soya and nuts this was a turning point in her life and the main reason to write this book in the first place. To face up to challenges of not being able to include any gluten, dairy, soya or nuts while cooking for her family, she knew she needed to formulate healthy diet and lifestyle changes that are sustainable, practical and achievable.

In this book Nada combines her scientific knowledge and culinary enthusiasm to show how food free from dairy, gluten, soya and nuts can be wonderfully tasty, easily prepared as well as nutritionally balanced.

First published in 2015 by New Holland Publishers Pty Ltd

London • Sydney • Auckland

The Chandlery Unit 9, 50 Westminster Bridge Road, London SE1 7QY, United Kingdom

1/66 Gibbes Street, Chatswood, NSW 2067, Australia

5/39 Woodside Ave, Northcote, Auckland 0627, New Zealand

www.newhollandpublishers.com

A record of this book is held at the British Library and the National Library of Australia.

ISBN: 9781742577524

Managing Director: Fiona Schultz

Publisher: Diane Ward

Editor: Holly Willsher

Designer: Kathie Baxter Eastway

Food Photography: Nada Farina

Production Director: Olga Dementiev

Printer: Toppan Leefung Printing Limited

10 9 8 7 6 5 4 3 2 1

All details have been updated and to best of publisher knowledge all restaurants have been contacted and recipe information is correct.

Keep up with New Holland Publishers on Facebook

www.facebook.com/NewHollandPublishers